Eosinophils in Asthma

Proceedings of a Symposium held at
Lucerne, Switzerland, December 1987

PERSPECTIVES IN ASTHMA · 4

Eosinophils in Asthma

Edited by

J. MORLEY
Pharmaceutical Division,
Sandoz Ltd,
Basel,
Switzerland

and

I. COLDITZ
CSIRO,
Division of Animal Health,
NSW, Australia

ACADEMIC PRESS
Harcourt Brace Jovanovich, Publishers
London San Diego New York Berkeley Boston Sydney Tokyo Toronto

ACADEMIC PRESS LIMITED
24/28 Oval Road
LONDON NW1 7DX

United States Edition published by
ACADEMIC PRESS INC.
San Diego, CA 92101

British Library Cataloguing in Publication Data is available

ISBN-0-12-506452-7

Typeset by Eta Services (Typesetters) Limited, Beccles, Suffolk
Printed in Great Britain by St Edmundsbury Press Limited, Bury St Edmunds, Suffolk

Contents

Preface

The first studies of autopsy material in asthma revealed a prominent eosinophilia within the lung tissue of asthmatics. Subsequent studies have consistently confirmed this phenomenon; none the less, little attention has been devoted to the role of this cell in the pathogenesis of asthma. Neglect of eosinophils was inevitable, once it had been recognized that there is an association between lung eosinophilia and the incidence of mast cells. Over the last two to three decades, mast cell activation has dominated the majority of schemes proposed to account for asthma pathogenesis. This imbalance has been compounded by placing eosinophils in a subordinate role, following suggestion that these cells nullify certain consequences of mast cell activation.

A number of factors have brought eosinophils back into prominence. First, the constituents of eosinophil granules have been characterized chemically and biologically and shown to be highly toxic materials. Secondly, it has been established that eosinophils generate substantial amounts of peptidoleukotrienes and of PAF, which acts as a selective stimulus to intrapulmonary accumulation and activation of eosinophils. Thirdly, progressive clarification of the chemical structure and biological properties of lymphokines has revealed that these materials control not only the proliferation and maturation of eosinophils, but the activation of these cells. Finally, studies of the effect of established anti-asthma drugs have revealed that several are able markedly to diminish migration of eosinophils into lung tissues.

In order to review these developments, a two-day meeting was held in Lucerne, Switzerland in December 1987. The format of the meeting favoured extensive discussion, which was recorded and transcribed for inclusion in this publication together with manuscripts covering each presentation. One participant was unable to provide a manuscript, which has necessitated substitution by an abstract in order to avoid an inordinate delay between presentation and publication. It is hoped that this volume will be appreciated as a contribution to the reinstatement of eosinophilia as an important element in asthma.

J. Morley   Basel
I. Colditz   May, 1989

List of Contributors

D.K. Agrawal Allergic Disease Center, Creighton University School of Medicine, 2500 California Street, Omaha, Nebraska 68178, USA

S. Aoki Preclinical Research, Sandoz AG, CH 4002 Basel, Switzerland

K. Boubekeur Preclinical Research, Sandoz AG, CH 4002 Basel, Switzerland

P.L.B. Bruijnzeel Schweizerisches Institut fur Allergie und Asthmaforschung (SIAF), Obere Strasse 22, CH 7270 Davod-Plats, Switzerland

A. Capron The Johns Hopkins University of Medicine, Clinical Immunology Division, Baltimore, Md, USA

M. Capron Centre d'Immunologie et de Biologie Parasitaire, Unité Mixte INSERM U167-CNRS 624, Institut Pasteur, 1 Rue du Pr A. Calmette, 59019, Lille Cédex, France

A. Champion Department of Allergy and Clinical Immunology, Cardiothoracic Institute, London, UK

J. Chihara 4th Department Internal Medicine, Kinki University School of Medicine, Onohigashi, Osakasayama, Osaka 589, Japan

I. Clark-Lewis The Biomedical Research Centre, University of Columbia, Vancouver, D6T 1W5, Canada

I. Colditz   CSIRO, Division of Animal Health, Armidale 2350, NSW, Australia

O. Cromwell   Department of Allergy and Clinical Immunology, Cardiothoracic Institute, London, UK

J.G.R. de Monchy   State University Hospital, Department of Allergology, Groningen, The Netherlands

A.J. Frew   Department of Allergy and Clinical Immunology, Cardiothoracic Institute, London, UK

T. Fukuda   Department of Allergy & Immunology, Dokkyo University School of Medicine, Tochigi 321-02, Japan

G.J. Gleich   Department of Internal Medicine and Immunology, Division of Allergic Diseases, Mayo Medical School, Mayo Clinic and Foundation, Rochester, MN 55905, USA

A. Hartnell   Department of Allergy and Clinical Immunology, National Heart and Lung Institute, Dovehouse Street, London SW3 6LY, UK

H.F. Kauffman   State University Hospital, Department of Allergology, Groningen, The Netherlands

A.B. Kay   Department of Allergy and Clinical Immunology, National Heart and Lung Institute, Dovehouse Street, London SW3 6LY, UK

E. Kloprogge   State University Hospital, Department of Allergology, Groningen, The Netherlands

K. Kurihara   Department of Allergy and Clinical Immunology, Cardiothoracic Institute, London, UK

C. Leprevost   Centre d'Immunologie et de Biologie Parasitaire, Unité Mixte INSERM U167-CNRS 624, Institut Pasteur de Lille, France

A.F. Lopez   Division of Human Immunology, Institute of Medical and Veterinary Science, Frome Road, Adelaide, South Australia 5000

S. MacDonald   Centre d'Immunologie et de Biologie Parasitaire, Unité Mixte INSERM U167-CNRS 624, Institut Pasteur de Lille, France

S. Makino   Department of Allergy and Immunology, Dokkyo University School of Medicine, Tochigi 321-02, Japan

T. Miyamoto   Department of Medicine & Physical Therapy, Faculty of Medicine, University of Tokyo, Japan

R. Moqbel   Department of Allergy and Clinical Immunology, Cardiothoracic Institute, London, UK

J. Morley   Preclinical Research, Sandoz AG, CH 4002 Basel, Switzerland

S. Motojima   Department of Medicine & Clinical Immunology, Dokkyo University School of Medicine, Mibu, Tochigi, 321-02 Japan

S. Nakajima   4th Department Internal Medicine, Kinki University School of Medicine, Onohigashi Osakasayama, Osaka 589, Japan

H. Okudaira, Department of Medicine & Physical Therapy, Faculty of Medicine, University of Tokyo, Japan

C.G.B. Peterson   The Laboratory for Inflammation Research, Department of Clinical Chemistry, University Hospital, S-751 85 Uppsala, Sweden

L. Prin   Centre d'Immunologie et de Biologie Parasitaire, Unité Mixte INSERM U167-CNRS 624, Institut Pasteur de Lille, France

C.J. Sanderson   National Institute for Medical Research, The Ridgeway, Mill Hill, London NW7 1AA, UK

S. Sanjar   Preclinical Research, Sandoz AG, CH 4002 Basel, Switzerland

M.F. Shannon   Division of Human Immunology, Institute of Medical and Veterinary Science, Frome Road, Adelaide, South Australia 5000

T. Shida   Sagamihara National Hospital, Center for Rheumatology and Allergy, Japan

C.J.F. Spry   Department of Immunology, St George's Hospital Medical School, Cranmer Terrace, London SW17 0RE, UK

M. Suko   Department of Medicine & Physical Therapy, Faculty of Medicine, University of Tokyo, Japan

P.-C. Tai   Department of Immunology, St George's Hospital Medical School, Cranmer Terrace, London SW17 0RE, UK

N. Tamura   Allergic Disease Center, Creighton University School of Medicine, 2500 California Street, Omaha, Nebraska 68178, USA

Y. Terashi   Department of Medicine & Clinical Immunology, Dokkyo University School of Medicine, Mibu, Tochigi, 321-02 Japan

M. Tomassini   Centre d'Immunologie et de Biologie Parasitaire, Unité Mixte INSERM U167-CNRS 624, Institut Pasteur de Lille, France

G. Torpier   Centre d'Immunologie et de Biologie Parasitaire, Unité Mixte INSERM U167-CNRS 624, Institut Pasteur de Lille, France

R.G. Townley, Allergic Disease Center, Creighton University School of Medicine, 2500 California Street, Omaha, Nebraska 68178, USA

M.A. Vadas   Division of Human Immunology, Institute of Medical and Veterinary Science, Frome Road, Adelaide, South Australia 5000

P. Venge   The Laboratory for Inflammation Research, Department of Clinical Chemistry, University Hospital, S-751 85 Uppsala, Sweden

J. Verhagen   Department of Pulmonary Disease, University Hospital, Catharijnesingel 101, NL-3511 CG Utrecht, The Netherlands

G.M. Walsh   Department of Allergy and Clinical Immunology, Cardiothoracic Institute, London, UK

A.J. Wardlaw   Department of Allergy and Clinical Immunology, Cardiothoracic Institute, London, UK

S.I. Wasserman   University of California, Medical Centre, San Diego, CA 92103, USA

T. Yukawa   Department of Medicine and Clinical Immunology, Dokkyo University School of Medicine, Mibu, Tochigi, 321-02 Japan

1

Regulation of Eosinophilopoiesis in Man

M. A. Vadas, A. F. Lopez, M. F. Shannon and I. Clark-Lewis*

Division of Human Immunology
Institute of Medical and Veterinary Science
Frome Road, Adelaide, South Australia, 5000

*The Biomedical Research Centre
University of British Columbia
Vancouver, D6T 1W5, Canada

1.1 INTRODUCTION

Since the time of Ehrlich eosinophilia has been one of the more readily recognizable clinical syndromes. Its presence has been associated with a number of disease states especially allergic and parasitic (1) but the association of blood and sputum eosinophilia with asthma has also been noted (2).

The observation by Metcalf and colleagues (3) that the production of blood cells from their bone marrow progenitors requires the presence of haemopoietic growth factors (HGF) (originally defined operationally as

Eosinophils in Asthma
ISBN 0-12-506452-7

Table 1   Properties of eosinophilopoietic cytokines

	Amino acid length	Chromosomal localization	Proliferating cells stimulated	Mature cells stimulated
IL-3[a]	133 (5)[b] predicted	5q31 (6)	M,[c] N, E, Ma, Mg, Mix, Ery (7–10)	E, not N (7)
GM-CSF	127 (11)	5q31 23–31 (12)	M, N, E, Mg, Mix, Ery (13, 14)	M, N, E (14, 17)
IL-5	115 (18, 19)	5q31 (20)	E (19, 21, 22)	E (21, 22)

[a]   Interleukin-3, IL-3; granulocyte-macrophage colony stimulating factor, GM-CSF; interleukin-5, IL-5.
[b]   Numbers in parenthesis are references supporting quoted data.
[c]   M = macrophage; E = eosinophil; Mg = megakaryocyte; Ery = erythroid; N = neutrophil; Ma = mast cell; Mix = mixed cell colony (includes capable of being repeated, the *in vitro* equivalent of progenitor cells).

colony stimulating factors—CSFs) has suggested that it is an excess of some of these factors that results in the eosinophilia associated with disease. The important observations of Basten and Beeson (4), amply confirmed by others, that eosinophilia is largely a T cell dependent phenomenon further suggested that eosinophilopoietic growth factors originate from T lymphocytes.

1.2   THE THREE EOSINOPHILOPOIETIC GROWTH FACTORS

Over the past four years human factors have been cloned that can give rise to the production of eosinophils in cultures of bone marrow. The important properties are summarized in Table 1. Several key points should be emphasized.

1.2.1   Apparent Redundancy

There is an *apparent redundancy* in the system. Why should three and not one factor be involved in eosinophilopoiesis? The explanation is not yet known but the following possibilities exist:

1. different factors work in different *micro-environments*; IL-5 may be primarily involved in peripheral eosinophil activation, whilst IL-3 in bone marrow haemopoiesis;
2. different factors are involved in steady state bone marrow production and

Table 2   Synergistic effect of rhGM-CSF and rhG-CSF in enhancing O_2-production by human neutrophils stimulated by 10^{-7} M FMLP

GM-CSF (ng/ml)	G-CSF (COS cell dilution)		
	α	1/60	1/6
0	4.2[a]	5.5	7.8
1	5.6	6.6	11.1
10	6.6	7.6	9.4
100	7.3	8.3	11.1

Human neutrophils were pre-incubated for 45 min at 37°C with different concentrations of rhGM-CSF, rhG-CSF or medium control and then stimulated with 10^{-7} M FMLP for 15 min at 37°C in the presence of cytochrome-c (12.4 mg/ml). O_2-production was measured by the reduction of cytochrome -C using an extinction coefficient of 21.1 nm.
[a] Mean of triplicate determinations. Standard expressed as nmoles of $O_2^-/10^6$ neutrophils, deviations were less than 15% of mean. No combination of CSFs released O_2^- without FMLP.

in conditions when there is *selective eosinophilia*; thus IL-3, and to a lesser extent GM-CSF, will give rise to many lineages and may be involved in steady state haemopoiesis. In allergy or parasitism with selective eosinophilia IL-5 might be elaborated. IL-5 only affects eosinophils and is the only cytokine that could give rise to this clinical picture;

3. maximum responses require *synergism* between the factors. Synergism might be seen in proliferative responses and clear evidence exists for this in mice as pre-incubation of bone marrow cells with IL-3 substantially increases (at least tenfold) the eosinophilopoietic response to IL-5 (23). Also in primates *in vivo*, IL-3 allowed a strong eosinophilopoietic response to small doses of GM-CSF which by themselves were ineffective (24). It can be anticipated that synergism will also be seen in eosinophil activation. In the case of neutrophils, this type of synergism has been seen in the mouse between G-CSF and GM-CSF (25) and also takes place in the human (Table 2), but no evidence for eosinophils is available.

1.2.2   Chromosomal Localization

Each HGF is the product of a single gene, and all three are located on band q23-31 of chromosome 5. The genes for IL-3 and GM-CSF have been mapped to within 9 Kb of one another (23) but the exact position of IL-5 is not yet known. The close localization of these genes is remarkable and suggests common evolutionary roots.

Table 3   Range of functions stimulated in eosinophils by eosinophilopoietic cytokines

Function	Cytokines		
	IL-3	GM-CSF	IL-5
Survival	—	+ (16,29,30)	+ (29)
ADCC (tumour)	+ (7)	+ (15,16)	+ (22)
ADCC (Schistosomula)	—	+ (31,34)	—
O_2-generation	+ (7)	+ (16,35,36)	+ (22)
Phagocytosis	+ (7)	+ (7,16)	+ (22)
LTC_4-generation	—	+ (34)	—
Chemotaxis	—	+ (37,38)	—
Adherence	+ (39)	+ (39)	+ (39)
Degranulation	—	—	—
Modulation of surface antigens	—	+ (16,40)	+ (21)

Plus sign indicates evidence supporting stimulation of function. References are given in parenthesis. Dash indicates lack of evidence on those points.

1.2.3   Cellular Sources

The spectrum of HGF secreted by different cells differs and is subject to modulation. There is evidence for such a situation in mice where, even among T cells, different subsets give rise to different spectra of haemopoietic growth factors (27) and given clones of T cells secrete their own, relatively fixed, set of factors (28). There is clear evidence that some T cells can elaborate all three eosinophilopoietins. Given the different spectrum of action of these molecules it appears important to have an instructional model which allows the transcription of all three, or any two, or any one of these HGFs to be initiated depending on the circumstances. This problem will be addressed later.

1.3   EOSINOPHIL ACTIVATION

Another important property of HGFs is their capacity to activate the function of mature cells. The spectrum of functions stimulated by HGF on eosinophils is broad (Table 3) and may underlie the capacity of eosinophils to damage tissues, a property central in the pathogenesis of asthma. In hypereosinophilic syndromes there is an association between hypogranular (degranulated?) eosinophils and endomyocardial damage (41). Surprisingly, the ability of eosinophil growth factors to induce eosinophil degranulation has so far received very little attention.

IL-3, GM-CSF and IL-5 are all able to activate eosinophil function (Table

Table 4 Stimulation of antibody-dependent eosinophil-mediated cytotoxicity by eosinophilopoietic cytokines

	% Cytotoxicity[a]
Nil	0
Mock transfected COS cells supernatant	7 ± 1[b]
IL-3[c]	18 ± 3
GM-CSF	30 ± 2
IL-5	21 ± 3

[a] Effector: target ratio of 30:1.
[b] Arithmetic mean 1 ± SEM of triplicate determinations. Eosinophils were 94% pure after passing buffy coat cells through a discontinuous metrizamide gradient (42).
[c] Cloned cytokines were used either in the purified form (GM-CSF) or as a COS cell supernatant (IL-3 and IL-5). The appropriate controls are nil and mock transfected COS cell supernatant respectively.

4) but their relative potency or the relative spectrum of their activity has not yet been fully determined. Interestingly in comparing the activation of function between neutrophils and eosinophils several differences emerge:

1. the *magnitude of activation* of eosinophils is always greater than that of neutrophils; this may reflect the lower background of eosinophils or that neutrophils are already partially activated, but still suggests that the presence or absence of these factors is a critical determinant of eosinophil function;
2. whilst HGFs are capable of priming neutrophils to respond better to exogeneous ligands such as f-Met-Leu-Phe in the capacity to generate O_2^-, on eosinophils these factors have a *direct effect* in raising production of O_2^- (7, 35, 36). This may be an important determinant in understanding why, in certain cases of eosinophilia, a great amount of vessel damage is seen.

The hypothesized pathogenic role of eosinophils has highlighted the potential usefulness of antagonists that could prevent the secretion or function of eosinophilopoietins. In order to develop such antagonists we have embarked on a series of experiments which attempt to understand the structure–function relationships of these factors and the regulation of transcription of their genes.

1.4 STRUCTURE–FUNCTION RELATIONSHIP OF GM-CSF

As a model eosinophilopoietin we chose GM-CSF and carried out structure–function studies in an effort to define critical parts of the molecule and to

Table 5   Effect of GM-CSF peptides on eosinophil generation and function

Parameter tested	GM-CSF peptides[a]			rhGM-none	
	1-127	14-127	25-127CSF[b]		
Eosinophil colonies[c]	71	56	0	62	0
ADCC[d]	**45.4**	**37.0**	17.0	**53.8**	22.4

[a] Chemically synthesized as described by Clark-Lewis et al. (43).
[b] 30 ng/ml rhGM-CSF.
[c] Number of eosinophil colonies from 5×10^4 non-adherent bone marrow cells plated per dish.
[d] Antibody-dependent eosinophil mediated cytotoxicity expressed as percentage of maximum killing (15) and performed in triplicate. Emboldened numbers differ from nil control by $p < 0.25$ or less.

generate specific antagonists. GM-CSF is a 127 amino acid protein with two disulphide bonds in the 1–3, 2–4 configuration. It has 53 aminoterminal residues before the first disulphide bond (54–96) and has six carboxyterminal residues after the second disulphide bond (87–121).

Our initial efforts used chemically synthesized molecules and truncations from the aminoterminus (43). Chemically synthesized hGM-CSF was an effective stimulus for eosinophil formation and activation. However, deletion of the 24 amino acids in the aminoterminus resulted in complete loss of activity. A summary (Table 5) shows that these peptides, like one consisting of amino acids 14–127, either retained all their function (including the stimulation of progenitor cells or mature cells) or, like amino acids 25–127, lost all their function. In no case was there a selective loss or retention of the capacity to stimulate eosinophils compared to neutrophils. Although these findings give clear indications for the active sites or GM-CSF they suggest that for selective antagonists of eosinophil production or activation similar studies will have to be performed on IL-5.

1.5   TRANSCRIPTIONAL REGULATION OF GM-CSF

The main inferred properties of HGF production, the capacity to be induced and their tissue specific production, could be explained at the level of transcriptional regulation. In general, gene transcription is thought to be regulated by proteins that bind to the promoter region of the gene in question and either enhance or repress the rate of transcription. These "DNA-binding proteins" are found, besides other places, in the nucleus of cells capable of

Table 6 Cellular distribution of nuclear-factor (NF) GMa and NF-GMb

Name	Cell line Probable origin	NF-GMa	NF-GMb
U5637	Bladder carcinoma	+ +	+ +
HUT78	T cell leukaemia	+ +	+ +
JURKAT	T cell leukaemia	+ +	+ +
HUT102	HTLV-I transformed T-cell	+ +	+
MLA144	Gibbon T cell leukaemia	+ +	−
LiBr	Melanoma	+ +	−
HL-60	Pro-myelocytic leukaemia	+ +	−
U937	Pro-monocytic leukaemia	+ +	−
SP2	Mouse myeloma	−	−
K562	Erythroleukaemia	−	−
47C7	T cell hybridoma	−	−

making the protein product from the gene in question. The capacity of these proteins to bind to DNA or to interact with the transcriptional machinery can be regulated by external agents, such as phorbol esters, that activate transcription (44).

We have previously described two nuclear factors in U5637 cells (NF-GMa and NF-GMb) that bind to two nucleotide sequences (cytokine (CK)-1 and CK-2) in the GM-CSF promoter, and inferred that these factors are important in the transcriptional regulation of GM-CSF (45). The cellular distribution of NF-GMa and NF-GMb is restricted (Table 6) and NF-GMb is induced by agents, leading to secretion of GM-CSF. These properties suggest an important role for these proteins in GM-CSF gene transcription.

1.6 HYPOTHESIS ON REGULATION OF EOSINOPHILOPOIESIS

Interestingly sequences similar to CK-1 are present in all eosinophilopoietic genes, GM-CSF, IL-3 and IL-5 (Table 7) and the possibility arises that the nuclear factor NF-GMa binds to all three. This can be tested by inhibition experiments in which the binding of NF-GMa to GM-CSF CK-1 is blocked by excess of cold CK-1 like sequences from IL-3, GM-CSF and IL-5, and could show that that same nuclear factor is involved in the regulation of all three genes. The strength of binding to the different CK-1 like sequences may in turn reflect the propensity to initiate transcription. Thus we would hypothesize that, under normal conditions, NF-GMa regulates a steady rate of production of an appropriate mixture of IL-3, GM-CSF and IL-5. Upon an allergic or parasitic challenge, a new protein "NF-IL-5", may be made which

Table 7   Cytokine-1 sequences of eosinophilopoietic factors

	Sequence	(Residue)	Sequence	(Residue)
IL-3	GAGGTTCCAT	(-126 to -117)	GAGATCCCAC	(-325 to -316)
GM-CSF	GAGATTCCAC	(-95 to -86)	GGGATTACAG	(-361 to -352)
IL-5	AAGATTCTTC	(-212 to -203)		

would bind other sequences in the IL-5 gene promoter. This leads to its enhanced transcriptional rate and thus gives greater levels of IL-5 as an absolute amount and in relation to the other HGFs.

Although this type of analysis is in its infancy, it will clearly be possible to test tissues for the presence of various nuclear factors which may give important indications of the pathogenesis of diseases. For example, certain leukaemic cells may show high levels of a given nuclear factor responsible for the continuous production of a haemopoietic growth factor on which the cells' growth depends. In the case of diseases associated with selective eosinophilia, such as some carcinomas of the lung and T cell lymphomas, the malignant cells may be producing high intrinsic levels or abnormal types of nuclear factors which bind to the promoter region of eosinophil growth factor genes, in general, and perhaps to IL-5 in particular.

1.7   SUMMARY

Eosinophilia can be caused by each of three haemopoietic growth factors (HGF), interleukin-3 (IL-3), granulocyte–macrophage colony stimulating factor (GM-CSF) and interleukin-5 (IL-5). These factors can also activate eosinophil function and thus the capacity of eosinophils to damage tissues.

Attempts at regulating eosinophil numbers or function will rely on specific antagonists of eosinophil-active HGFs or the selective inhibition of production of these cytokines. Structure–function studies and studies of transcriptional regulation of GM-CSF are presented as a model approach to these problems.

Acknowledgements

This work was supported by grants from the National Health and Medical

Research Council, Anti-Cancer Foundation of the Universities of South Australia and National Cancer Institute grant no. 1 RO1 CA45822-01.

REFERENCES

1. Beeson, P. B. and Bass, D. A. (1978). *In* "Major Problems in Internal Medicine" (Ed. L. H. Smith, Jr.), Ch. 14. W. B. Saunders, Philadelphia.
2. Horn, B. R., Robin, E. D., Theodore, J. and Kessel, A. V. (1976). *New Eng. J. Med.* **292**:1152–1155, 1976.
3. Metcalf, D. (1984). Elsevier/North Holland, Amsterdam, 1-486.
4. Basten, A. and Beeson, P. B. (1970). *J. Exp. Med.* **131**, 1288.
5. Yang, Y-C., Ciarletta, A. B., Temple, P. A., Chung, M. P., Kovacic, S., Witek-Giannotti, J. S., Leary, A. C., Kriz, R., Donahue, R. E., Wong, G. G. and Clark, S. C. (1986). *Cell* **47**, 3–10.
6. LeBeau, M. M., Epstein, N. D., O'Brien, S. J., Neinhuis, A. W., Yang, Y-C., Clark, S. C. and Rowley, J. D. (1987). *Proc. Natl. Acad, Sci. USA* **84**, 5913–5917.
7. Lopez, A. F., To, L. B., Yang, Y-C., Gamble, J. R., Shannan, M. F., Burns, G. F., Dyson, P. G., Juttner, C. A., Clark, S. and Vadas, M. A. (1987). *Proc. Natl. Acad. Sci. USA* **84**, 2761–2765.
8. Messner, H. A., Yamasaki, K., Jamal, N., Minden, M. M., Yang, Y-C., Wong, G. G. and Clark, S. C. (1987). *Proc. Natl. Acad. Sci. USA* **84**, 6765–6769.
9. Leary, A. G., Yang, Y-C., Clark, S. C., Gasson, J. C., Golde, D. W. and Ogawa, M. (1987). *Blood* **70**, 1343–1348.
10. Sieff, C. A., Niemeyer, C. M., Nathan, D. G., Ekern, S. C., Bieber, F. R., Yang, Y-C., Wong, G. and Clark, S. C. (1987). *J. Clin. Invest.* **80**, 818–823.
11. Wong, G. G., Witek, J. S., Temple, P. A., Wilkens, K. M., Leary, A. C., Luxenberg, D. P., Jones, S. S., Brown, E. L., Kay, R. M., Orr, E. C., Shoemaker, C., Golde, D. W., Kaufman, R. J., Hewick, R. M., Wang, E. A. and Clark, S. C. (1985). *Science* **228**, 810–815.
12. Huebner, K., Isobe, M., Croce, C. M., Golde, D. W., Kaufman, S. E. and Gasson, J. C. (1985). *Science* **230**, 1281–1285.
13. Sieff, C. A., Emerson, S. G., Donahue, R. E., Nathan, D. G., Wang, E. A., Wong, G. G. and Clark S. C. (1985). *Science* **230**, 1171–1173.
14. Metcalf, D., Begley, C. G., Johnson, G. R., Nicola, N. A., Vadas, M. A., Lopez, A. F., Williamson, D. J., Wong, G. G., Clark, S. C. and Wang, E. A. (1986). *Blood* **67**, 37–45.
15. Vadas, M. A., Nicola, N. and Metcalf, D. (1983). *J. Immunol.* **130**, 795–799.
16. Lopez, A. F., Williamson, D. J., Gamble, J. R., Begley, C. G., Harlan, J. M., Klebanoff, S. J., Waltersdorph, A., Wong, G., Clark, S. C. and Vadas, M. A. (1986). *J. Clin. Invest.* **78**, 1220–1228.
17. Grabstein, K. H. *et al.* (1986). *Science* **232**, 506–508.
18. Azuma, C., Tanabe, T. Konishi, M., Kinashi, T., Noma, T., Matsuda, F., Yoaita, Y., Takatsu, K., Hammarstrom, L., Edvard Smith, C. I., Severinson, E. and Honjo, T. (1986). *Nucleic Acids Research* **14**, 9149–9158.
19. Campbell, H. D., Tucker, W. Q. J., Hort, Y., Martinson, M. E., Mayo, G., Clutter-

buck, E. J., Sanderson, C. J. and Young, I. G. (1987). *Proc. Natl. Acad. Sci. USA* **84**, 6629.

20. Sutherland, G. R., Baker, E., Callen, D. F., Campbell, H. D., Young, I. G., Sanderson, C. J., Garson, O. M., Lopez, A. F. and Vadas, M. A. *Blood* (in press).

21. Lopez, A. F., Begley, C. G., Williamson, D. J., Warren, P. Vadas, M. A. and Sanderson, C. (1986). *J. Exp. Med.* **163**, 1085–1099.

22. Lopez, A. F., Sanderson, C. J., Gamble, J. R., Campbell, H. D., Young, I. G. and Vadas, M. A. (1988). *J. Exp. Med.* **167**, 219–224.

23. Warren, D. J. and Moore, M. A. S. (1988). *J. Immunol.* **140**, 94–99.

24. Donahue, R. E., Seehra, J., Norton, C., Turner, K., Metzger, M., Rock, B., Carbone, S., Seghal, R., Yang, Y. C. and Clark, S. C. (1987). *Amer. Soc. Hematology, Blood* **388**, 133a.

25. Lopez, A., Nicola, N., Burgess, A. W., Metcalf, D., Battye, F., Sewell, W. A. and Vadas, M. A. (1983). *J. Immunol.* **131**, 2983–2988.

26. Mossman, T. R., Cherwinski, H., Bond, M. W., Geidlin, M. A. and Coffman, R. A. (1986). *J. Immunol.* **136**, 2348.

27. Kurt-Jones, E. A., Hamberg, S., Ohara, J., Paul, W. E. and Abbas, A. K. (1987). *J. Exp. Med.* **166**, 1774–1787.

28. Kelso, A. and Metcalf, D. (1985). *J. Cell. Physiol.* **123**, 101.

29. Begley, C. G., Lopez, A. F., Nicola, N. A., Warren, D. J., Vadas, M. A., Sanderson, C. J. and Metcalf, D. (1986). *Blood* **68**, 162–166.

30. Owen, W. F., Rothenberg, M. E., Wilberstein, D. S., Gasson, J. C., Stevens, R. L., Austen, K. F. and Soberman, R. J. (1987). *J. Exp. Med.* **166**, 129–141.

31. Vadas, M. A., Dessein, A., Nicola, N. and David, J. R. (1981). *Aust. J. Exp. Biol. Med. Sci.* **59**, 739–741.

32. Dessein, A., Vadas, M. A., Nicola, N. A., Metcalf, D. and David, J. R. (1982). *J. Exp. Med.* **156**, 90–103.

33. Thorne, K. J. I., Richardson, B. A., Taverne, J., Williamson, D. J., Vadas, M. A. and Butterworth, A. E. (1986). *Eur. J. Immunol.* **16**, 1143–1149.

34. Silberstein, D. S., Owen, W. F., Gasson, J. C., DiPersio, J. F., Golde, D. W., Bina, J. C., Soberman, R., Austen, K. F. and David, J. R. (1986). *J. Immunol.* **137**, 3290–3294.

35. Vadas, M. A., Varigos, G., Nicola, N., Pincus, S., Dessein, A., Metcalf, D. and Battye, F. (1983). *Blood* **61**, 1232–1241.

36. Pincus, S., Dessein, A., Lenzi, H., Vadas, M. A. and David, J. R. (1984). *Cell. Immunol.* **87**, 424–433.

37. Wang, J. I., Collella, G., Allavena, P. and Mantovani, A. (1987). *Immunology* **60**, 439–444.

38. Vadas, M. A. (1983). *In* "Immunobiology of the Eosinophil" (Eds T. Yoshida and M. Torisu), 77–95. Elsevier, North Holland.

39. Vadas, M. A., Lopez, A. F., Gamble, J. R. and Shannon, M. F. *Progress in Leukocyte Biology* (in press).

40. Arnout, M. A., Wang, E. A., Clark, S. C. and Sieff, C. A. (1986). *J. Clin. Invest.* **78**, 597–601.

41. Spry, C. J., Weetman, A. P., Olsson, I., Tai, P. C. and Olsen, E. G. (1985). *Heart Vessels* **1**, 162–169.

42. Vadas, M. A., David, J. R., Butterworth, A. E., Pisani, N. T. and Siongok, T. A. (1979). *J. Immunol.* **122**, 1228.

43. Clark-Lewis, I., Lopez, A. F., Vadas, M., Schrader, J. W. and Kent, S. B. H. *In*

"Proceedings of the 5th International Lymphokine Workshop" (Ed. C. W. Pierce). Humma Press, Clifton, N.J. (in press).
44. Maniatis, T., Goodburn, S. and Fisher, J. A. (1987). *Science* **236**, 1237–1245.
45. Shannon, M. F., Gamble, J. R. and Vadas, M. A. (1988). *Proc. Natl. Acad. Sci. USA.* **85**, 674–678.

DISCUSSION

Kay (Chairman): You have spent most of the time talking about GM-CSF and pointed out that it was, as opposed to IL-3, oligopotential. Is there any information as to what is happening *in vivo*, in terms of the sequence of events which finally produce mature eosinophils? If there is not, would you like to speculate whether it is possible that these events might take place outside the bone marrow. You might, in a chronic eosinophil inflammatory state, be able to probe in some way, to see which colony-stimulating factors are actually being expressed. It is possible that cells may be talking to each other at the tissue level?

Vadas: As usual, your question is provocative and points to the actual knot of the problem, which is to work out what is happening *in vivo*. It is difficult to detect which cytokine is produced in a particular site. The only technology that really can do this is *in situ* hybridization to see whether a cell is making that particular message. We have spent about two years trying to do this; I think some other people have been more successful, but we haven't been able to get any *in situ* hybridization with cytokine genes which stand up to the relevant controls. So I think the problem is an important one, but I don't think that the technology at the moment is there to answer it. Now I'm going to hypothesize. I think there will be some cytokines that will be only made in the bone marrow which will be their normal dutiful role. There will be others that will be made in the periphery and will be primarily involved in mature cell activation in joints, in the lung, or other tissues in which inflammation takes place. Their primary role will be to cause granulocytes to live longer, to be more active, and to destroy bacteria. I think that whether the process is inflammation, an autoimmune response, or a reaction to bacterial products, the process will be exactly the same. You can detect some of these CSFs in the circulation under extreme conditions such as endotoxin shock.

Kay: The active site 18–24 is obviously of biological interest in the activation events that you describe; is this also the hot spot for stimulating eosinophil maturation?

Vadas: Absolutely. They are identical. You can do binding studies showing that inactive peptides don't compete for binding of the recombinant molecules and that active peptides do compete for the binding.

Suko: May I ask you two brief questions. Do you have any information about the effect of chemoattractants upon eosinophil maturation and differentiation?

Vadas: That's easy. No, I don't have any information on differentiation that is useful.

Suko: The second question. Do eosinophil progenitors exist in the blood circulation?

Vadas: They do and I think they exist in humans in surprisingly large numbers. Their role is not yet clear and it is not evident whether they have to localize to the bone marrow. My hypothesis, and I think that may be what lies behind your question, is that eosinophilopoiesis will be able to take place in sites of allergic inflammation, for example in the lung. Otherwise, I see no good reason for the circulation of large numbers of eosinophil progenitors, but I may be wrong.

Spry: Can I follow that up? I don't know of any evidence that eosinophils are made outside the bone marrow in man, unless you have some data that isn't published.

Kay: Has anybody actually looked really very critically at this issue? It is such an important question.

Spry: Yes, a lot of people have looked.

Vadas: But how have they looked?

Spry: All you have to do is to look for mitoses. It's very simple. It has been done for years.

Vadas: Well, I would submit that it's easy to miss.

Kay: It's rather a crude way of looking at the problem, isn't it? I mean, you could have a scenario where you wouldn't necessarily see massive mitosis, but you could have some sort of formation of granules which didn't involve frank cell division.

Vadas: I've looked at the data from hypersensitive lesions. A lot of mitosis is occurring there.

Spry: Not among the eosinophils. I don't think you need to worry about the site of mitosis. The marrow is a super place for making eosinophils. There is nothing wrong with it.

Vadas: We'll hypothesize like the number of angels on the head of a pin.

Kay: We should continue this discussion after the session. It is a very interesting point, but there are lots of questions.

Wasserman: To come back to that point for a second, we have looked at the differentiation of mast cells in the nasal passages. It is clear that there has been proliferation, but I don't think that mitosis has been easily recorded there either; so I think that mitosis is a rather insensitive way of determining proliferation. What those data suggest is that there is something crucial beyond the growth factors, namely the micro-environment of the tissue itself in the context of differential regulation. Cells do not see 20 000 units of GM-CSF in the absence of other growth factors. There is a family of growth factors, with which cells are interacting at a particular time, including factors generated locally that we've not yet learned about; such factors may or may not be secreted and may only be displayed on cell surfaces, as for example, upon fibroblast or endothelial cells. Locally generated factors are probably the major reason why the growth is so successful in the bone marrow and not in other tissues; the problem should not be viewed as a growth factor situation. This is more of an editorial than a question, but it is absolutely essential that we understand the growth factors, the active site, which cells make the factors, and in which tissues. Focusing only upon the growth factors is an approach that is too limited, don't you think? There is my question. Do you think growth factor is the entire answer?

Vadas: Again a very perceptive question. I think you are absolutely right. We know already a number of cytokines that critically inhibit the effect of, well not these growth factors, but certainly lymphocytic growth factors, an example of an inhibitory factor in TGF$_B$. It is the orchestration of these and the various proportions of factors that is important. I accept that you are right in a sense, but we can only do a certain amount. As long as one recognizes that what is being done is a drop in the ocean and does not cease from thinking what the ocean does. I'm sorry, if this is not a very good answer. Your question is a self-answering one.

Dahl: I would like to ask you if you had information on the kinetics of the production of these factors? Is it enough to have a short stimulus to induce production or do you have to have a long-lasting stimulus? I know that you can measure this by functional assays, but do you know anything about the functional half-life of the substances?

Vadas: We haven't done a lot ourselves because I know there are several other groups involved in study of the regulation of production. Vassali's group in Geneva and Seves in Boston have been able to show that certain phagocytic stimuli can trigger macrophages into production of these cytokines for a prolonged period. I would submit that they would be the best to answer this question. GM-CSF is produced and then turned off by itself, whereas tumour necrosis factor production is maintained for much longer. So each cytokine has its own set of rules in each cell type. If you go to endothelial cells you think you are going to find exactly the same thing; yet it is exactly the opposite. So, it's a hugely interesting complicated field. With respect to your second question, functional half-life is a bit of a funny thing. The affinity of CSF receptors is of the order of 10^{-12} molar. Although their circulating half-life has a phase 1 of 6 min and a phase 2 of about 30–40 min, they stick to the receptor and their biological effect is seen for days on end. This is why you can get away with subcutaneous injections because the receptors become saturated and store the information for quite a long time. So although CSF is eliminated from the circulation rapidly, a single injection can have a prolonged biological effect.

Spry: Matthew, I have a problem that I have been wrestling with for some years; I wonder if you could help me with it. Why aren't all granulocytes activated when they leave the bone marrow? If granulopoietic factors are also probably the major tissue activating stimuli, why haven't they got that property right from the start?

Vadas: You and I have the same problem and I think it really relates to the micro-environment as indicated by Steve Wasserman. We have several pieces of evidence to indicate that if you take calls that look identical from bone marrow and peripheral blood, they are quite different in their functional responsiveness. So I would think in the bone marrow there are other factors in operation, although I don't know what they are. These factors would prevent cell emigration until a certain stage of maturation had been reached and would inhibit cell functions; when these factors stop working, the cells can emigrate and be subject to the next set of regulatory phenomena.

Spry: One thought I have on this explanation is that granulocytes cross the endothelium twice in their life—once when they leave the bone marrow to get into the blood and then when they leave the blood to get into the tissues. It seems impossible that regulatory influences occur at those two crucial points since the endothelium is such a major site for growth factor production and activating factor production, unless movement in one direction inhibits the activation process and movement in the other stimulates it. It seems to me that thinking in this way could help.

Kay: Interesting points indeed and there are many possibilities not the least being that plasma proteins can somehow down regulate the activation process.

2

Mast Cells and Eosinophils

S. I. Wasserman

University of California, Medical Center
San Diego, CA 92103, USA

The association of eosinophilia with allergic disease has been known for nearly a century. Because of the central role of the mast cell in the genesis of allergic disease, workers nearly two decades ago began to investigate the association between mast cell activation and eosinophil production and accumulation. Initial work was directed towards the elucidation of factors generated by mast cells which affected the migration of eosinophils. Anaphylactic supernatants of animal and human lung tissue sensitized with IgE and challenged with specific antigen were demonstrated to contain materials which induce the migration of eosinophils across millipore barriers. Physicochemical characterization of these low molecular weight factors revealed them to be heat stable and to possess molecular weights of 300–500 daltons. The ability to isolate mast cells of the rodent led to the identification of the fact that these low molecular weight factors were preformed and present in the mast cell granule of rodents. They were packaged along with histamine and other mast cell mediators, and could be released from their mast cell stores upon activation of the cell through immunologic or non-immunologic

Eosinophils in Asthma
ISBN 0-12-506452-7

mechanisms. Further analysis of factors generated by rodent mast cells which could attract eosinophils demonstrated that, not only were there low molecular weight materials termed eosinophil chemotactic factor of anaphylaxis, but also molecules of 1–3000 molecular weight, peptide in nature, which were also preformed and released upon immunologic challenge. As techniques were developed to isolate human lung mast cells, they, too, were demonstrated to possess within their granules materials chemoattractant for eosinophils which were released upon IgE-mediated activation of this cell. Further analysis of mast cell activation in the human led to the identification of low molecular weight eosinophil chemoattractants released into the circulation of patients experiencing allergic disorders. In this regard, humans suffering from antigen induced bronchoprovocation reactions and physical urticaria, particularly cold urticaria, were demonstrated to possess, within their circulation, factors which induced the directed migration of eosinophils. Isolation of the materials from plasma of patients with cold urticaria revealed a family of low molecular weight eosinophil attractants. These factors were separated by gel filtration, ion exchange and high-pressure liquid chromatography, and revealed three different molecules: the highly acidic hydrophobic low molecular weight factor consistent with ECF-A, and two higher molecular weight materials which differed in their hydrophobicity and acidity. All of these factors attracted eosinophils directly. In addition to these low molecular weight preformed materials, it has also been demonstrated that histamine and platelet activating factor are capable of affecting eosinophil migration. Histamine is a rather non-specific and impotent chemoattractant which, at high concentrations, inhibits eosinophil-directed migration. Platelet-activating factor, on the other hand, is an exceptionally potent chemoattractant for eosinophils which is active both *in vitro* in attracting eosinophils across millipore filters, and *in vivo* where its instillation via the tracheal bronchial tree or intravenously leads to rapid accumulation of eosinophils within the airway. In addition to attracting eosinophils, mast cells generate products which activate this unique polymorphonuclear leukocyte target cell population. For example, ECF-A augments eosinophil production of platelet-activating factor. This interrelationship between mast cells and eosinophils has obvious implications for the genesis and expression of allergic disease, and forms an important unexplored territory for therapeutic intervention in allergic diseases.

DISCUSSION

Kay (Chairman): I would like to remind those of you who are old enough to remember, and I shouldn't think there are many of you here, that this ECF-A story goes back now almost 15 years. Very briefly, as Dr Wasserman said, I was largely responsible for bringing to people's attention that the anaphylactic effusate from human and guinea-pig lung stimulated with homocytotropic antibody, or IgE in the human system, did contain activity which seemed preferentially to attract eosinophils. This was confined to the low molecular region of between approximately 500 and 1000 daltons. Certainly in the guinea-pigs, eosinophils elicitated by horse serum were far more active than neutrophils elicitated by glycogen stimulation. The preferential activity in human blood was less marked but seemed to favour the eosinophil, but this really is pretty ancient history. I think it was you Steven, who afterwards showed that comparable activity could be extracted from mast cells and lung by freezing and thawing, suggesting that this was a preformed mediator. Subsequently Dr Goetz and Dr Austin published a paper in 1974 saying that most of this activity could be attributed to two tetrapeptides val-gly-ser-glu and ala-gly-ser-glu. I think a lot of people had great difficulty in showing that these synthetic peptides have chemotactic activity which approached that of the crude or partially refined anaphylactic effusate. I think that we really have been hung up on this point ever since and I don't think that anybody involved in the use of chemotactic assays, including myself, has ever been able to show that these two peptides really have appreciable activity in a test of chemotaxis. They do, like many peptides, increase eosinophil adhesiveness, as you showed in one of our rosette assays. That may be an area where they have a role although even that is far from clear. What has become apparent over the last few years is that the activity of these peptides is quite insignificant compared to platelet-activating factor (PAF). I think that this slide demonstrates the contrast quite well. You can see that the activity of PAF is really quite considerable, whereas histamine and the peptides are pretty pathetic. In that situation, the responses to peptides were only just above controls; in other experiments, you can show that there are twice or two-and-a-half times that of control, but compared to PAF, these chemotactic responses are negligible. Hence, what we were looking at in 1972 was largely PAF; I'm sure that until we prove otherwise, that is what it was.

If I could just briefly indulge you for another moment with the next slide, please. It is interesting that it is very difficult to show an association between lymphocyte-derived materials and eosinophil chemotaxis. You see the migration response to PAF over three concentrations but to a range of recombinant cytokines there is really no eosinophil chemotactic activity. I'm sure Dr Sanderson won't mind me mentioning that he also has given me some of his IL-5. We haven't tested it over the right dose range, he tells me; but, at very high concentrations, it doesn't seem to work. We have to do more work on IL-5, over a much wider dose range. The next slide gives the rank order of eosinophil chemotactic factor activities, PAF, C5a, C5a des arg, LTB_4, fMLP and MNCF. These latter materials have activity, but it doesn't approach that of PAF. The concentrations are high merely because I'm giving you the optimal concentration above which you begin to see high dose inhibition. As Steven said, LTB_4 really is very weak when compared to PAF, C5a and C5a des arg.

I am still not convinced that the mast cell was contributing appreciably to the chemotactic activity that we were observing from the chopped lung fragments. I think one could still entertain the possibility that the activity could be derived from other cells bearing the low-affinity IgE receptors and that the association between mast cells and eosinophils is getting weaker rather than stronger in terms of eosinophil chemotaxis signals released from mast cells. That is a bit provocative for you, Steven, but there are popular misconceptions which must be challenged. One is that IgE is working exclusively through mast cells in those late phase skin models. The other thing which has muddied the field considerably is the popular misconception that cromoglycate is predominantly a mast cell stabilizer; I think many of us have showed clearly that this just isn't so in humans. So, a little controversy Steven, but I'm sure that is something you will respond to.

Wasserman: I don't know where to begin. To start with, our experiences with chemoattraction and the panel of chemoattractant mediators which I demonstrated, is very similar to yours. Our data are less quantitative, but I would agree with you that PAF and C5a are the two most potent chemotactic activities directed to eosinophils and that the tetrapeptides of the ECF-A are extremely unimpressive chemoattractants. I think there are families of low molecular weight materials which can be found in blood. One can extract materials from mast cells which have chemoattractant potential and whether they are the most important or not remains to be seen. I think your comments are provocative but not easily answered, because we don't know who is doing what to whom. I think that as we develop better biochemical techniques for isolating mediators, particularly from complex biological tissues and fluids, and as we develop the assays for *in situ* hybridization in order to understand what cell is where and what cell has what properties, we can get an answer to these questions.

My point of view is that IgE, mast cells and eosinophils are interrelated somehow but we don't yet understand this relationship. Maybe the inter-relationship is at a higher level and mast cells come along with these eosino-phils no matter what we do, because they respond to very similar stimuli. Perhaps the mast cell–eosinophil interaction is relatively minor and it is the stimulation from up above by lymphocytes, fibroblasts, nerve growth factor or whatever, that stimulates both of these. I think it's of great interest that these cell types possess many overlapping properties (leukotriene C_4, PAF) and many different factors, some of which may complement one another, others which compete. Heparin for example can bind to a lot of the basic materials released from eosinophils. I think that the crucial thing is not to worry about who said what first, or which cell is the most important, but rather to try and finally to get to the answer of which cell is doing what. I agree with you completely that people who hold positions that "my mole-cule" or "my cell" is the important one have hampered developments in this area more than they have helped. I think now we are finally at the stage where we understand that IgE can activate a variety of cells and this is a stimulus to investigation in this area.

Kay: I do agree, probably the strongest link is at the IL-3 level at this point in time.

Wasserman: To be provocative I think IL-3 is probably a vastly overrated and unimportant molecule in the human. I think that there are many others, such as IL-5 and maybe IL-9, that are maybe more important.

Gleich: You question the relationship between mast cell product and eosino-phil chemotaxis. It is almost dogma; the medical students read it in their first introductory texts, but I think there is reason to be somewhat sceptical about that. On the other hand, it seems to me that it is difficult to ignore the data that one sees in these late phase reactions. We've studied extensively the IgE-mediated late phase reactions in skin and recently have applied the same pro-cedures to lung. It is clear that in normal skin there are mast cells but there are essentially no eosinophils and relatively very few neutrophils. A few minutes after initiation of an IgE-mediated reaction in the skin either provoked directly in a sensitized person or induced passively in someone as a PK reaction, there is a minimal cell migration. This occurs within 15 min to an hour; what one does see is just profound eosinophil degranulation and equally strikingly a neutrophil degranulation as evidenced by deposition of neutrophil elastase. In that context, it seems to me difficult to ignore the underlying importance or presumed importance of the mast cell. One looks at the skin before the reaction and mast cells are there. We know the mast cells have receptors for IgE. How do you get around that train of logic?

Kay: Quite simply. At the risk of being repetitive, the point is that there are other cells in addition to mast cells, which can respond to this anti-IgE stimulus.

Wasserman: But how about codeine? One of the things you can show is that compound 48–80 or codeine can also induce eosinophil accumulation. Presumably these materials do not interact with these other cells.

Kay: Well, you don't know.

Wasserman: No, we don't know. Nor do you know that the fact that IgE can interact with other cells provides an explanation. All that we know is that there are multiple potential explanations for what we see and that we shouldn't get too committed to any particular one. But I agree that we shouldn't throw the baby out with the bath water, that there is going to be a relationship between the mast cell and the eosinophil which will persist after we've worked through the lymphokines and after we've worked through the low affinity IgE receptor. It will come out, the answer will be developed.

Vargaftig: I would like to come back to the PAF story. A few years ago we tried to find PAF in the perfusate from challenged guinea-pig lungs and we failed to do so when the challenge was via the artery, which is the usual route. The Wellcome group could find a lot of PAF and a lot of lyso-PAF, the inactive metabolite, when they challenged by an intratracheal route. So apparently there is an alveolar component. One hypothesis might be the alveolar macrophage was releasing PAF. Connected to this are some data for *in vivo* eosinophilic infiltration in lungs and, in our laboratory, we could demonstrate a very marked eosinophil infiltration when guinea-pigs were injected intravenously either with PAF or antigen. This infiltrate followed within 6–24 hours and, very interestingly, was blocked by PAF antagonists not only when the effect was due to PAF, but also when allergen was the stimulus to accumulation. So two chemically unrelated PAF antagonists blocked eosinophil infiltration *in vivo* induced by antigen or PAF itself. Two other manoeuvres achieved the same effect, both of which ultimately deplete platelets. When you administer either anti-platelet antiserum or prostacyclin, eosinophil infiltration, examined after 24 h, was completely suppressed.

If I may make a last comment, I would like to make a plea to use actively sensitized animals whenever we are testing a potential agonist. We have experiments now in press, in which the pharmacology of an isolated lung obtained from a naive animal or from a passively sensitized animal is completely different from an animal that is actively sensitized. Very interestingly, a lot of histamine is released by arachidonic acid, by leukotriene D_4 and by PAF itself providing a lung comes from a sensitized animal whereas a naive lung or a passively sensitized lung doesn't release histamine at all. So, there is a sort of a turning off and turning on of the lung in association with sensitisation. We are hypothesizing that, during immunizaton, these lungs are invaded by inflammatory cells; there are about 40% more eosinophils in the pre-shocked lung.

Kay: Your observations on PAF induced eosinophilia are very interesting and you made the point in your article that it is the atopic individual who seems to recruit the eosinophil.

Vargaftig: Yes, that is in human skin. Here, I am referring to the guinea-pig lung. These observations fit very well together.

Kay: In that skin model, Paul Atkins and others have shown a substantial PAF release during the late phase of the IgE-mediated skin reaction. It is difficult for me to see the mast cell as the source of such impressive concentrations of PAF. But, anyway, I mustn't air my prejudices too much. I am impressed, I must say, with the data on PAF-induced eosinophilia, its inhibition and the kinetics as they relate to eosinophil infiltration.

Wasserman: There are a few points that have to be addressed. I think it is clear that actively sensitized animals are going to differ from passively sensitized animals. They will have experienced the generation of T cell products that are going to change everything. That is the strongest evidence for the fact that these cytokines are important. One has to be careful when using animal models. The guinea-pig is an extremely eosinophil-prone animal and the fact that certain factors work or don't work, and certain other constituents activate or don't activate, may be extremely interesting. However, it may not be relevant to human disease and I think that that is always a very important consideration. Finally, I don't think that the fact that large amounts of PAF come out late in the skin reaction means that the mast cell is not important at the onset of the allergic reaction. The massive accumulation of PAF in a skin blister 4 and 6 h later may reflect the fact that the eosinophils come into the lesion and then make PAF.

   The crucial issue is what started the reaction. The data that Dr Vargaftig just referred to indicate that sensitization, which arms the mast cells, is one way to get things going; but this isn't the full answer. Sensitizing the lymphocytes is another answer. However, I don't know of any systems in which there are no mast cells, which would provide a way to start answering this question. We need to breed animals that lack mast cells; I don't think the W/W^v mouse is a mast cell deficient animal but it is a mast cell granule deficient animal which is another story all together. I don't think we have the ability yet to answer this question in a definitive manner.

Kay: Thank you very much Stephen. I think there is one thing we are agreed on. There are still a lot of questions which need answering in this system, even after this length of time.

Sanjar: Just one comment I would like to make about the relationship between the mast cell and the eosinophils. You said yourself that a β-adrenoceptor agonist could inhibit the early response, but not the late response. We know that the β-adrenoceptor agonist drugs are the most potent mast cell stabilizing agents known, in both human and guinea-pig. It therefore seems that inhibition of mast cell activation is not really important for the development of the late-phase asthmatic response.

Wasserman: So mast cell stabilizers have been defined on the basis of their ability to prevent histamine release?

Kay: Well, that depends on the model system employed.

Wasserman: I think that it is true that these drugs are mast cell stabilizing agents in the sense of degranulation. In other systems though, this may not apply. For example, in the rodent you cannot demonstrate any effect of β-adrenergic drugs on mast cell function.

Kay: Well now, this is a very good point; in humans you can. Salbutamol has a much more potent mast cell stabilizing effect than cromoglycate. Salbutamol blocks the early asthmatic response. It blocks the early rise in histamine release and has no effect on the late phase, so I think it is quite a strong argument.

Dahl: I would like to hear your opinion today about the work or opinions of previous years about the interaction between mast cell constituents and eosinophil constituents. The theory was that you had this interaction for inactivation, and to provide regulation between the cells. The other thing I would like to know relates to the many studies of *in vitro* chemotaxis using chambers. Do you know if there are any studies which show that it is possible to deduce from these *in vitro* observations what is occurring *in vivo* in humans? Also is the status of the donor important in chemotaxis studies. We have made skin studies, using skin chambers in a similar way to Dr Gleich. Exposure to LTB_4 produced a very weak chemoattractant effect upon neutrophils and eosinophils. This observation prompts me to raise the issue, because you found very high chemotactic activity of LTB_4 for neutrophils *in vitro* and scarcely any activity for eosinophils.

Wasserman: The last one first. I don't think there is a very good correlation between *in vitro* chemoattraction and *in vivo* chemoattraction. Certainly a number of these inflammatory drugs or inflammatory compounds have been studied *in vivo*. PAF, leukotriene B_4 and FMLP have been injected into a variety of tissues in a range of species, where potency in neutrophil accumulation has been demonstrated. LTB_4, C5a and PAF in skin or in hamster cheek pouch have shown profound neutrophil accumulation. In some systems PAF has also caused eosinophil accumulation, when given intravenously or into the airway, but not when injected into the skin; in the skin, you primarily see neutrophils. That is my experience.

Kay: I'm sure that Dr Vargaftig would like to respond to that.

Vargaftig: If you take a normal patient you find neutrophils but if you take an allergic patient you find mostly eosinophils; one-third of the cells are eosinophils and one-third of this fraction is degranulated.

Wasserman: I do think that the donor is crucial. I think the donor was crucial to the identification of the tetrapeptides as having any chemoattractant activity and I think the donor is obviously going to be crucial for the expression of chemotactic potency. What we have seen is that the cutaneous responsiveness in atopic individuals is very different than that in normal individuals. This may have to do with the pre-arming of a whole variety of cell types. However, I think that one cannot take literally what you see in a Boyden chamber and translate it to the human. In addition, when you make blisters or other manoeuvres, you have to contend with all the inactivating, regulatory and counter-regulatory processes occurring in blood, serum or in association with cells. So I think that the answer is not available.

Kay: I think that it's worth mentioning, Stephen, that these peptides were not prepared from dispersed mast cells and did not even involve an immunologic stimulus. They were prepared from whole lung fragments which were chopped up, frozen and thawed. It was the most crude mixture imaginable. And, futhermore, the lipid fraction was thrown away; there had been a pre-conception that the active principle was a peptide and hence that component was progressively purified.

Wasserman: Well, the peptide principle was based on data that you accumu-lated showing that protease treatment decreased the amount of chemoattrac-tant activity. That could have been, but there is a trivial explanation, namely that many of these proteases bind lipids and could have removed the PAF. Don't get me wrong; I do not defend that data at all; I'm not part of that paper and I didn't do any of that work and I'm not an apologist for the ECF tetrapeptides. To answer your other question Dr Dahl about the relative action of mast cells vis-a-vis eosinophils. I think that one can look at them as pro-inflammatory and anti-inflammatory interactions. Certainly the eosino-phil contains constituents which can dampen mast cell function. They have histaminase and they have heparin. Mast cell histamine can be inactivated by eosinophils and eosinophilic major basic protein can bind to mast cell heparin. This may operate at low levels of activation, such as occur in normal people on a day-to-day basis where mast cells are being activated minimally and when the eosinophil and the mast cell reside next to each other. I think it is still a sustainable hypothesis that mast cells and eosinophils dampen each other as well as activate each other. I think it is clear from the work of Dr Gleich and others that, in the disease state, when large numbers of eosino-phils are present, the interaction is not a protective one.

3

Control of Eosinophil Production

C. J. Sanderson

National Institute for Medical Research,
The Ridgeway, Mill Hill, London, NW7 1AA, UK

3.1 INTRODUCTION

Normal individuals have very small numbers of eosinophils, but this can change dramatically so that they become the predominant leukocyte. The best known examples of diseases associated with eosinophilia are allergic reactions and infections by helminths. This ability to produce large numbers of eosinophils in response to external stimuli provides an interesting example of the control of haemopoiesis.

The possibility that the control of eosinophilia is mediated by a lymphokine was initially suggested by the T cell dependence of eosinophilia induced by parasites in rats (1) and by observations that supernatants of activated spleen cells can induce eosinophil colony formation (2). For these reasons we sought to identify the activity produced by mouse T cells which was stimulating eosinophil production *in vitro*, and have used experimental infection of mice by the cestode *Mesocestoides corti* to induce eosinophilia. The activity

Eosinophils in Asthma
ISBN 0-12-506452-7

identified was named eosinophil differentiation factor (EDF) and the term interleukin-5 (IL-5) has become accepted for this factor.

Although no human equivalent had been characterized, the identification and subsequent cloning of the murine factor led to the cloning and expression of the analogous human factor. The availability of both human and mouse IL-5 is an important step towards understanding the control of eosinophilia.

3.2   ASSAYS FOR EOSINOPHIL PRODUCTION

In our hands the liquid culture system has been more sensitive than the colony assay system for assaying mouse eosinophil production *in vitro* and, furthermore, has been more adaptable for the handling of large numbers of samples. In the human system both the colony assay and liquid culture systems can be used, although the time of assay is much longer than in the mouse.

3.2.1   Mouse Culture Systems

In preliminary experiments it was found that the addition of crude spleen cell supernatants to liquid bone marrow cultures (3) caused a significant production of eosinophils, and the numbers of eosinophils were markedly increased when the bone marrow was taken from mice undergoing eosinophilia as the result of experimental parasite infection (4). To facilitate the handling of large numbers of samples, a microplate adaptation of these cultures was developed. At first the eosinophils produced in each well were estimated by counting total cells in a Coulter Counter, followed by differential staining to determine the percentage. While it was important initially to quantify the assay in this way, the technique is extremely laborious and so experiments were carried out to test assay for peroxidase as an indirect assay for eosinophils. Apart from neutrophils which produce myeloperoxidase, this enzyme is not produced in significant amounts by other mammalian cells. It was shown that the production of eosinophils could be estimated indirectly by assaying for eosinophil peroxidase using *o*-phenylenediamine. In murine cultures this provides a specific assay for eosinophils, even in the presence of large numbers of neutrophils (5, 6). The reason for this appears to be the relatively low levels of myeloperoxidase in mouse neutrophils.

The apparent low sensitivity of the eosinophil colony assay has no clear explanation for while under optimal culture conditions eosinophil colonies can be obtained (7), we have not found the expected relationship between colony numbers and potential to produce eosinophils in liquid culture. While the paucity of eosinophil colonies in mouse colony assays may be due to trivial factors such as fetal calf serum and agar batches, the same conditions give rise to expected numbers of neutrophil and macrophage colonies. Furthermore, the same culture conditions and, indeed, the same murine EDF, used with human bone marrow give rise to appreciable numbers of eosinophil colonies (8). The practical implication of this problem is that most of our work has been based on the liquid culture system, where it is not possible to quantify directly the number of eosinophil progenitor cells.

3.2.2 Human Culture Systems

In human marrow cultures both the liquid and colony assay systems can be used as assay systems (6, 8). However, assay for eosinophil peroxidase is not specific as neutrophils in human bone marrow cultures have significant levels of myeloperoxidase. Furthermore, in our hands, there is no sufficiently accurate method for discriminating between myeloperoxidase and eosinophil peroxidase by the use of inhibitors, so that use of the peroxidase assay is very limited. The colony assay cultures are incubated for 14 days, when the semisolid culture medium is removed to a microscope slide, dried and stained, so that individual colonies can be identified. Although the liquid culture system also requires at least 14 days incubation, the determination of eosinophil numbers by differential counting is less laborious than counting colonies, and so this assay system is preferred. When assaying EDF in the absence of other haemopoietic factors, as for example during the purification of EDF, it is possible to use the peroxidase assay system provided the cultures are incubated for 21 days. The longer culture time allows a decline in the number of neutrophils, so that eosinophils are determined against a low peroxidase background.

3.3 MURINE IL-5

3.3.1 Identification

Following the development of the assay system, a panel of T cell clones were tested for the production of EDF and other lymphokines. A high proportion produced an activity which stimulated eosinophil differentiation. Coordinate analysis, of the activity produced by individual T cell clones in each of the assays suggested that the eosinophil differentiation activity was distinct from IL-2 and IL-3. This was confirmed by gel filtration of supernatant from one of these clones (NIMP-T2, after further expansion in culture). The EDF separated with a peak M_r of 45 000, and was thus clearly distinct from IL-3 and GM-CSF (9).

A series of T cell hybrids was produced by fusing spleen cells from *M. corti* infected mice to the T lymphoma BW5147. These were tested for their ability to produce EDF after stimulation with phorbol myristate acetate (PMA) and one selected that produced high levels of EDF. After repeated selection by subcloning this hybrid (NIMP-TH1) produced high levels of EDF but none of the other lymphokines for which it was tested (10). This provided a source of EDF for biological, biochemical and molecular investigation.

3.3.2   Biochemical Characterization

EDF from both a T cell clone (NIMP-T2) and the hybrid NIMP-TH1 appeared after gel filtration as a wide band ranging from M_r 32 000 to 62 000 with a peak at 46 000 (9). The activity was destroyed by trypsin and bound to immobilized lentil lectin, suggesting it was a glycoprotein. When the cells were grown in the presence of tunicamycin to block N-linked glycosylation, the activity produced, eluted with a M_r of 30 000 indicating a maximum size for the protein and suggesting that the carbohydrate was not essential for biological activity.

3.3.3   cDNA Cloning

A cDNA expression library was produced from NIMP-TH1 mRNA and screened by expression in COS cells. A clone (pEDFM-4) which expressed EDF activity was isolated from this library and the insert was found to be 653 bp in length. A second clone was isolated from the library by hybridization (pEDFM-5) and this contained an insert of 1534 bp (11). Both clones code for a single open reading frame of 133 amino acids and are identical to the sequence reported for T cell replacing factor/B cell growth factor II (TRF/BCGFII) (12), thus confirming our original report that EDF and BCGFII were properties of a single molecule (see Section 3.8.1).

3.4   GENE STRUCTURE

A mouse EDF cDNA coding region fragment was used as a probe for Southern blotting and isolation of the mouse and human genes. Mouse and human genomic lambda libraries were prepared and screened with the mouse probe. Phages from hybridizing plaques were purified from each library, and sub-cloned for sequencing. A 3.2 kb human fragment was inserted into the eukaryotic expression vector pcEXV-3 to give pEDFH-1 (13). This has the EDF gene in the same orientation as the SV40 early promoter in the vector, and expresses human EDF following transfection into COS cells, demonstrating that the complete coding region was present.

The nucleotide sequences of a 6.7 kb region spanning the mouse EDF gene (12) and of the 3.2 kb fragment containing the human EDF gene (13) were determined. The four exons of the genes were readily assigned by comparison with the cDNA sequence. The first two introns of the mouse gene are significantly longer than those in the human gene. The relative positions of the introns within the coding regions are identical in the two genes and all introns begin with GT and end in AG. A potential TATA box is located 20 bp (human) and 30 bp (mouse) upstream from the start of transcription, and there is at least one potential CAAT box around 80 bp upstream of the start of each gene. The 3' untranslated region of the mouse gene carries an additional segment of 738 bases just after the termination codon, giving rise to a mouse EDF mRNA which is much larger than its human counterpart. Apart from this, the exons are highly conserved.

Comparison of the mouse EDF gene sequence with murine genes encoding other haemopoietic growth factors did not reveal significant homology, with the exception of a region upstream of the TATA boxes of the EDF and granu-locyte-macrophage-CSF (GM-CSF) genes. This sequence is also present in the same position in the human EDF and GM-CSF genes. Similar sequences are present immediately upstream from the TATA boxes of some other lymphokine genes (14).

The human IL-5 gene is located at 5q31 and is deleted in patients with the 5q-syndrome (15). Both IL-3 (16) and GM-CSF (17) genes have been located to the same region of this chromosome. It has been established that the murine IL-3 and GM-CSF genes lie close together on mouse chromosome 11 (18) and it has been found that the murine IL-5 gene is also present on chromosome 11 (Campbell et al., in preparation). The genes encoding these three factors (as well as IL-4, although the chromosome location of this has not yet been published) share an overall structural similarity with similar exon sizes.

3.5 PROTEIN STRUCTURE

The genes encode EDF precursors of 133 amino acids in the mouse and 134 in humans. The predicted site of cleavage of the signal peptide is after amino acid 18 in the mouse and 19 in humans to give a processed protein of 115 amino acids in each case (M_r of 13 299 in the mouse and 13 149 in the human). As discussed above, the native mouse protein appears to be M_r of approximately 30 000 in non-glycosylated form, and so is likely to be a dimer. There are three potential N-glycosylation sites in the mouse EDF, the first and last of which are conserved in the human protein. Two cysteine residues are present in each mature protein at corresponding positions. There is 67% amino acid sequence identity between mouse and human EDF, this compares with 29% between mouse and human IL-3 and 52% between mouse and human GM-CSF.

3.6   BIOLOGICAL ACTIVITY OF IL-5

3.6.1   In Mice

As discussed above, adding EDF to mouse bone marrow cultures causes the production of eosinophils. A feature of this culture system is the relatively transient production of eosinophils compared to neutrophils, and the increased production of eosinophils when the bone marrow is taken from parasitized mice. The long-term production of neutrophils appears to be due to the maintenance of stem cell proliferation and the continued production of neutrophil precursors (3). It appears, therefore, that a similar production of eosinophil precursors is not occurring *in vitro*, even in the presence of EDF. Taken together, these factors suggest that EDF in these cultures is active only on precursor cells which are pre-committed to the eosinophil lineage and which are presumed to be increased as a result of the parasite infection.

To investigate the biological role of EDF in the production of eosinophilia *in vivo*, assays were carried out at different times after infection with *M. corti*. The development of eosinophilia in these infected mice is preceded by detectable levels of EDF in the serum. No IL-3 could be detected in serum samples at any stage of the infection (19). On gel filtration this serum EDF fractionated as a broad band with a peak at M_r 38 000, which is not dissimilar to EDF produced *in vitro*. This detection of EDF in serum is good evidence for a biological role of this factor in the development of eosinophilia.

3.6.2   In Humans

Eosinophil colony stimulating activity had been reported in conditioned media of various human cells or tissues containing mixed colony stimulating factors (CFS) (20) and this had led to the concept of an eosinophil-CSF (Eo-CSF). However, no such factor had been unequivocally identified and characterized. The situation was made more complex when purified human GM-CSF was shown to stimulate eosinophil colony formation (21). Thus at least some of the Eo-CSF activity in the crude conditioned media could have been due to GM-CSF. On the other hand it had been reported that crude murine spleen conditioned medium stimulated the production of eosinophil colonies in human bone marrow culture, and it was known that murine GM-CSF did not have activity in humans (22). It was therefore of interest to test purified murine EDF (mEDF) for activity in human cultures. The result was quite clear, murine EDF was found to stimulate the production of human eosinophil colonies, with negligible effect on other colony types (7).

This study of mEDF on human cells made a number of important points. Clone transfer experiments and the linear relationship between the number of bone marrow cells plated and colonies produced confirmed that the action of mEDF was directly on eosinophil progenitor cells. Furthermore, mEDF was found to induce similar numbers of colonies as sources of GM-CSF suggesting that the two factors were active on the same population of precursors. Thus it seemed likely that a human analogue and corresponding receptor for murine EDF must exist. Furthermore, the cross-species activity suggested that the two factors would show high sequence homology.

The cross-species activity made several studies with human eosinophils possible. In a study with peripheral blood eosinophils it was shown that mEDF increased their capacity to kill antibody-coated tumour cells, and to phagocytose serum opsonized yeast cells. This functional activation was associated with the enhanced expression of several surface antigens (7). mEDF had no effect on the functional activity of neutrophils. This work added to the growing list of factors capable of activating these cells in short-term functional assays. In another study, mEDF prolonged the survival of human peripheral blood eosinophils, but had no activity on the survival of neutrophils (23). This was shown to be a quick and sensitive assay for EDF and other CSFs.

3.7   ACTIVITY OF EOSINOPHILS PRODUCED IN CULTURE

3.7.1   Studies on Mouse Eosinophils

In bone marrow cultures EDF caused a significant production of eosinophils, with no increase in other cell types. Cultures containing bone marrow from mice infected with *M. corti* produced at least tenfold the number of eosinophils, as bone marrow from normal mice. At peak production the cultures from infected mice contained about 80–90% eosinophils (9). Under both the light and the electron microscope these were typical eosinophils, although the nuclear structure indicated that only a minority were fully mature. Functional studies for cytotoxic activity towards antibody-coated erythrocytes, demonstrated that like eosinophils taken from mice, they had receptors for IgG1, IgG2a and IgG2b, but not IgM, IgA or IgE (4, 9). These culture-derived eosinophils also killed schistosomula of *Schistosoma mansoni* in the presence of antibody and complement (9). It is therefore apparent that the culture system allows the differentiation of eosinophils to full functional maturity.

3.7.2   Studies on Human Eosinophils

Murine EDF or rhEDF can be used to produce functional eosinophils in human liquid bone marrow cultures (8, 13). Although there is considerable variation between marrow cells from different individuals, significant numbers of eosinophils appeared after about 2 weeks and reached a peak between 3 and 4 weeks. Until the third week most of the eosinophils were typical myelocytes, progressively developing into metamyelocytes. By about 6 or 7 weeks most of the cells were mature eosinophils. The eosinophils including the immature myelocytes were capable of killing antibody-coated tumour cells.

3.8   ACTIVITY ON B CELLS

3.8.1   Mouse B Cells

In the early 1970s experiments were carried out to produce antibodies in spleen cell cultures, and several different groups found that T cells could be removed from the cultures and replaced by T cell supernatants. The activity in these supernatants became known as T cell replacing factor (TRF) and was demonstrated to be of high molecular weight (24). Later, B cell growth factor II (BCGFII) was identified as a factor stimulating B cell proliferation in the presence of the co-stimulator dextran sulphate, and this factor was found to induce proliferation of the mouse B cell line BCL_1 (25). This factor was also found to be of high molecular weight.

As part of an analysis of lymphokine production by a panel of T cell clones, it was found that there was a high correlation between EDF activity and activity detected by the BCL_1 B cell tumour (26, 27). It was then found that these two activities co-purified through to a single band on polyacrylamide gel electrophoresis (26). Taken together, these results suggested that the two activities were the property of a single molecule. At about this time it was shown that purified TRF had BCGFII activity (28). Thus TRF, BCGFII and EDF were all properties of a single molecule.

On mouse B cells, *in vitro* IL-5 increases both proliferation and differentiation of pre-activated B cells to increase the number of cells producing immunoglobulin. Thus large B cells isolated from the spleen give much higher numbers of IgM and IgG antibody-producing cells in the presence of IL-5 than in control cultures (29). This large effect on IgM production by otherwise unstimulated B cells has been confirmed with unfractionated spleen cells (30). Furthermore, this work showed that, in the presence of bacterial lipopolysaccharide, there is an increase in IgA as well as IgM and IgG. However, the effect on IgA appears to be much less than the effect on IgM or IgG.

3.8.2   Failure to Detect Activity on Human B Cells

There have been a number of reports of human B cell growth factors of high molecular weight (BCGF-H) (31, 32). Because of the high molecular weight of mouse IL-5 and its activity as BCGFII and TRF, human IL-5 was clearly a candidate for some or all of these activities. The availability of rhIL-5 made it possible to test for BCGF activity. These experiments initially concentrated on the standard co-stimulator assays that had been used to identify BCGF in humans. Surprisingly, the hIL-5 was negative in these assays. It was therefore important not only to broaden the types of assay used, but also because of other activities which might potentially exist in COS cell supernatants, to use purified material of high biological activity.

This material was found not to have inhibitory activity in a B cell assay using commercially available low molecular weight BCGF (BCGF-L) (33), even at a dilution of 1:10, which represents approximately 8000 EDF units. It was active on the mouse BCL_1 cell line, but in none of the following human B cell assay systems (34). In each assay the rhIL-5 was tested over a wide range of dilutions up to a concentration of 1:50 (i.e. 1600 EDF units).

1. Proliferation assays with tonsillar or splenic B cells in the presence of the

co-stimulators anti-μ or PMA. This is the assay system most commonly used to identify human BCGF, and is analogous to the co-stimulator assay used to identify murine BCGFII. Although BCGF-L gave a positive result in all the assays, the hIL-5 was negative.

2. A restimulation assay in which tonsillar B cells are first activated with either SAC or a mixture of PDB and Ionomycin, or splenic B cells are first activated with anti-μ. Although human IL-4 gave a positive response, hIL-5 was negative.

3. Human IL-5 did not increase production of IgG or IgM by tonsillar B cells in a restimulation assay with SAC or PMA, nor did it increase IgG production by the Epstein–Barr virus transformed B lymphoblastoid CESS cell line.

4. Although either BCGF-L or IL-2 were able to stimulate proliferation of chronic lymphocytic leukaemia (B-CLL) cells freshly explanted from three different patients, rhIL-5 had no activity. Furthermore, although BCGF-L stimulated proliferation of the B lymphoma (L4) cell line and the mature B cell (HFB1) line, rhIL-5 had no activity.

5. Finally, because mIL-5 is active as a TRF, rhIL-5 was tested for its ability to replace T cells in specific antibody responses. Again rhIL-5 was negative in this system, with no increase in IgM, IgG or IgA antibody.

It seems likely therefore that hIL-5 does not have activity analogous to mouse BCGFII or TRF. Thus the BCGF-H (31, 32) are not likely to represent native forms of IL-5. Another possibility is that BCGF-L which is active in the same types of co-stimulator assays as mouse BCGFII/TRF represents the native form of IL-5, however, this material has no activity as an EDF. Final confirmation of this point must await the availability of highly active recombinant BCGF-L.

While these results clearly demonstrate that hIL-5 does not have activities analogous to mouse BCGFII or TRF, it does not rule out the possibility that this factor does have some other activity on human B cells. Two reports of IL-5 activity on human B cells exist (30, 35), but neither used purified material. In both cases it is difficult to evaluate the data because no statistical analysis is presented, and in one case the preparation of B cells contained a significant number of T cells (35).

3.9 CONCLUSION

IL-5 is an eosinophil differentiation and activating factor. It is specific for the eosinophil lineage in haemopoiesis, and is analogous to the CSFs described for other myeloid lineages. Some support for a biological role for this factor in the induction of eosinophilia comes from its appearance in the serum of mice during eosinophilia induced by a parasitic infection. Despite this we are still a long way from understanding the control of eosinophilia, and there may be other haemopoietic growth factors involved. The identification of IL-5 has made possible the production of functional eosinophils from both human and mouse bone marrow *in vitro*. A considerable amount of work is yet to be done before the full potential of this development can be realized.

The biological role of IL-5 as a B cell growth factor is unclear. In mice this activity is readily detectable *in vitro*. Although IgE antibody is associated with eosinophilia, current evidence indicates that IL-4 rather than IL-5 is active in IgE induction. IL-5 appears to increase production of IgM and to a lesser extent IgG and IgA antibody *in vitro*. In contrast to the mouse, human IL-5 does not appear to be active in analogous human BCGF assays.

The high conservation of the human and mouse IL-5 sequence in comparison with some of the other lymphokines is intriguing in relation to evolution. It is possible that selection favoured the conservation of IL-5 because of the importance of eosinophils in increasing resistance to metazoan parasites. We are therefore left with the paradoxical situation, that eosinophils may provide an important positive role in infectious disease, but leave the legacy of a negative role in non-infectious diseases such as hypersensitivity.

REFERENCES

1. Basten, A. and Beeson, P. B. (1970). Mechanism of eosinophilia. II Role of the lymphocyte. *J. Exp. Med.* **131**, 1288.
2. Metcalf, D., Parker, J. W., Chester, H. M. and Kincade, P. W. (1974). Formation of eosinophilic-like granulocytic colonies by mouse bone marrow cells *in vitro*. *J. Cell, Physiol.* **84**, 275.
3. Dexter, T. M., Allen, T. D. and Lajtha, L. G. (1977). Conditions controlling the proliferation of haemopoietic stem cells *in vitro*. *J. Cell. Physiol.* **91**, 335.
4. Strath, M. and Sanderson, C. J. (1985). The production and functional properties of eosinophils from bone marrow cultures. *J. Cell. Sci.* **74**, 207.
5. Strath, M., Warren, D. J. and Sanderson, C. J. (1985). Detection of eosinophils using an eosinophil peroxidase assay. Its use as an assay for eosinophil differentiation factors. *J. Immunol. Methods* **83**, 209–215.
6. Strath, M., Clutterbuck, E. J. and Sanderson, C. J. (1989). Production of human and murine eosinophils *in vitro* and assay for eosinophil differentation factors. *In* "Methods in Molecular Biology", Vol. 5, "Tissue Culture" (Eds J. Walker and J. W. Pollard). Humana Press Inc., Clifton, New Jersey.
7. Lopez, A. F., Begley, C. G., Williamson, D. J., Warren, D. J., Vadas, M. A. and

Sanderson, C. J. (1986). Murine eosinophil differentiation factor: An eosinophil-specific colony-stimulating factor with activity for human cells. *J. Exp. Med.* **163**, 1085.

8. Clutterbuck, E. J. and Sanderson, C. J. (1988). Human eosinophil production *in vitro* studied by means of murine eosinophil differentiation factor (IL5). *Blood* **71**, 646

9. Sanderson, C. J., Warren, D. J. and Strath, M. (1985). Identification of a lymphokine that stimulates eosinophil differentiation *in vitro*. Its relationship to IL3, and functional properties of eosinophils produced in cultures. *J. Exp. Med.* **162**, 60.

10. Warren, D. J. and Sanderson, C. J. (1985). Production of a T cell hybrid producing a lymphokine stimulating eosinophil differentiation. *Immunology* **54**, 615.

11. Campbell, H. D., Sanderson, C. J., Wang, Y., Hort, Y., Martinson, M. E., Tucker, W. Q. J., Stellwagen, A., Strath, M. and Young I. G. (1988). Isolation, structure and expression of cDNA and genomic clones for murine eosinophil differentiation factor. Comparison with other eosinophilopoietic lymphokines and identity with Interleukin-5. *Eur. J. Biochem.* **174**, 345

12. Kinashi, T., Harada, N., Severinson, E., Tanabe, T., Sideras, P., Konishi, M., Azuma, C., Tominaga, A., Bergstedt-Lindqvist, S., Takahashi, M., Matsuda, F., Yaoita, Y., Takatsu, K. and Honjo, T. (1986). Cloning of a complementary DNA encoding T-cell replacing factor and identity with B-cell growth factor II. *Nature* **324**, 70.

13. Campbell, H. J., Tucker, W. Q. J., Hort, Y., Martinson, M. E., Mayo, G., Clutterbuck, E. J., Sanderson, C. J. and Young I. G. (1987). Molecular cloning, nucleotide sequence, and expression of the gene encoding human eosinophil differentiation factor (interleukin 5). *Proc. Natl. Acad. Sci. USA* **84**, 6629.

14. Sanderson, C. J., Campbell, H. D. and Young, I. G. (1988). Molecular and cellular biology of eosinophil differentiation factor (Interleukin-5) and its effects on human and mouse B cells. *Immunological Reviews* **102**, 29

15. Sutherland, G.R., Baker, E., Callen, D. F., Campbell, H. D., Young, I. G., Sanderson, C. J., Garson, O. M., Lopez, A. F. and Vadas, M. A. (1987). Interleukin-5 is at 5q31 and is deleted in the 5q-syndrome. *Blood* **71**, 1150

16. Le Beau, M. M., Epstein, N. D. O'Brien, S. J., Nienhuis, A. W., Yang, Y-C., Clark, S. C. and Rowley, J. D. (1987). The interleukin-3 is located on human chromosome 5 and is deleted in myeloid leukemias with a deletion of 5q. *Proc. Natl. Acad. Sci. USA* **84**, 5913.

17. Huebner, K., Isobe, M., Croce, C. M., Golde, D. W., Kaufman, S. E. and Gasson, J. C. (1985). The human gene encoding GM-CSF is at 5q21–q32, the chromosome region deleted in the 5q-anomaly. *Science* **230**, 1282.

18. Barlow, D. P., Bucan, M., Lehrach, H., Hogan, B. L. M. and Gough, N. M. (1987). Close genetic and physical linkage between the murine haemopoietic growth factor genes GM-CSF and multi-CSF (IL3). *EMBO J.* **6**, 617.

19. Strath, M. and Sanderson, C. J. (1986). Detection of eosinophil differentiation factor and its relationship to eosinophilia in *Mesocestoides corti*-infected mice. *Exp. Hematol.* **14**, 16.

20. Nicola, N. A., Metcalf, D., Johnson, G. R. and Burgess, A. W. (1979). Separation of functionally distinct human granulocyte-macrophage colony stimulating factors. *Blood* **54**, 614.

21. Dao, C., Metcalf, D. and Bilski-Pasquier, G. (1977). Eosinophil and neutrophil colony forming cells in culture. *Blood* **50**, 833.

22. Metcalf, D., Cutler, R. L. and Nicola, N. A. (1983). Selective stimulation by mouse spleen conditioned medium of human eosinophil colony formation. *Blood* **61**, 999.
23. Begley, C. G., Lopez, A. F., Nicola, N. A., Warren, D. J. and Sanderson, C. J. (1986). Purified colony stimulating factors enhance the survival of human neutrophils and eosinophils *in vitro*: A rapid and sensitive microassay for colony stimulating factors. *Blood* **68**, 162.
24. Schimpl, A. and Wecker, E. (1975). A third signal in B cell activation by TRF. *Transpl. Rev.* **23**, 176.
25. Swain, S. and Dutton, R. W. (1982). Production of a cell growth promoting activity, (DL)BCGF, from a cloned T cell line and its assay on the BCL$_1$ B cell tumor. *J. Exp. Med.* **156**, 1821.
26. Sanderson, C. J., O'Garra, A., Warren, D. J. and Klaus, G. G. B. (1986). Eosinophil differentiation factor also has B cell growth factor activity. Proposed name interleukin 4. *Proc. Natl. Acad. Sci. USA* **83**, 437.
27. Sanderson, C. J., Strath, M., Warren, D. J., O'Garra, A. and Kirkwood, T. B. L. (1985). The production of lymphokines by primary alloreactive T cell clones. A co-ordinate analysis of 233 clones in seven lymphokine assays. *Immunology* **56**, 575.
28. Harada, N., Kikuchi, Y., Tominaga, A., Takaki, S. and Takatsu, K. (1985). BCGFII activity on activated B cells of a purified murine T cell replacing factor (TRF) from a T cell hybridoma (B151K12). *J. Immunol.* **134**, 3944.
29. O'Garra, A., Warren, D. J., Holman, M., Popham, A.M., Sanderson, C.J. and Klaus, G. G. B. (1986). Interleukin 4 (B cell growth factor II/eosinophil differentiation factor) is a mitogen and differentiation factor for preactivated murine B lymphocytes. *Proc. Natl. Acad. Sci. USA* **83**, 5228.
30. Yokata, T., Coffman, R. L., Hagiwara, H., Rennick, D. M., Takebe, Y., Yokata, K., Gemmell, L., Shrader, B., Yang, G., Meyerson, P., Luh, J., Hoy, P., Pene, J., Briere, F., Spits, H., Banchereau, J., de Vries, J., Lee, F. D., Arai, N. and Arai, K. (1987). Isolation and characterisation of lymphokine cDNA clones encoding mouse and human IgA enhancing factor and eosinophil colony stimulating factor activities: Relationship to interleukin 5. *Proc. Natl. Acad. Sci. USA* **84**, 7388.
31. Yoshizaki, K., Nakagawa, T., Fukunaga, K., Tseng, L. T., Yamamura, Y. and Kishimoto, T. (1984). Isolation and characterization of B cell differentiation factor (BCDF) secreted from a human lymphoblastoid cell line. *J. Immunol.* **132**, 2948.
32. Ambrus, J. L., Jurgensen, C. H., Brown, E. J. and Fauci, A. S. (1985). Purification to homogeneity of a high molecular weight human B cell growth factor; demonstration of specific binding to activated B cells; and development of a monoclonal antibody to the factor. *J. Exp. Med.* **162**, 1319.
33. Maizel, A. L., Sahasrabuddhe, S., Mehta, S.R., Morgan, L., Lachman, L. and Ford, R. (1982). Biochemical separation of human B cell mitogenic factor. *Proc. Natl. Acad. Sci. USA* **79**, 5998.
34. Clutterbuck, E. J., Shields, J., Gordon, J., Smith, S. H., Boyd, A., Callard, R. E., Campbell, H. D., Young, I. G. and Sanderson, C. J. (1987). Recombinant human interleukin-5 (IL5) is an eosinophil differentiation factor but has no activity in standard human B cell growth factor assays. *Eur. J. Immunol.* **17**, 1743.
35. Azuma, C., Tanabe, T., Konishi, M., Noma, T., Matsuda, F., Yaoita, Y., Takatsu, K., Hammerstrom, L., Smith, C.I.E., Severinson, E. and Honjo, T. (1986). Cloning of cDNA for human T cell replacing factor (interleukin-5) and comparison with the murine homologue. *Nucleic Acids Res.* **14**, 9149.

DISCUSSION

Kay (Chairman): Your work on IL-5 is clearly a landmark and a milestone in eosinophil biology. You spent quite a lot of your time distancing IL-5 from B cell growth factor II and have pointed to the difficulties of using the mouse antibody systems. I wonder if you could either tell us, or speculate, about the relationship between IL-5 and IgE production?

Sanderson: Had this material been active in any of the human B cell assays, we would have a nice assay system for human IL-5, rather than having to rely upon the colony assay, which is a tedious assay system. When we first saw the correlation between BCGFII and EDF in the mouse we thought, this may be the missing link; this is why we see IgE in eosinophilia. However, that seems not to be the case. IL-4 seems to be more important in the IgE response and Bill Paul's lab in NIH have done some very beautiful experiments demonstrating, both *in vitro* and *in vivo*, that IL-4 is very important. For example, using monoclonal antibodies, they could actually block the IgE response in a parasite infected mouse. So I think we must assume that IL-5 is not the primary stimulus for IgE production. Now in the mouse, BCGFII (IL-5) seems to be an IgA inducing factor. I emphasize that this applies in the mouse because I don't think the data in man are yet good enough to stand up to critical analysis; in the mouse there is no doubt about it. You do get IgA; that has been shown by several different laboratories even before the factor was cloned. Now the interesting thing is, if this factor is important in IgA production, how do you get an antibody response in the absence of eosinophilia? That is one of the central questions to be addressed. These biological cross-reactivities lead you to expect that, whenever you see one activity, you must always see the other. Yet, IgA and eosinophils have not been linked so closely. I don't understand why that should be so. That isn't to say that I don't believe in it; I merely don't understand it yet. I think there is more work to be done.

Vadas: I would like to say how much I enjoyed the talk. My question relates to your findings of cultures in the human where you had eosinophils of various degrees of maturity. It is partly a philosophical question because we think of granulocytes as end cells, unlike monocytes and macrophages which are capable of dedifferentiation. But that does raise the question whether a granulated cell can actually revert to an activated stage that you see earlier in a culture and whether our concept of any eosinophil as a mature end cell will have to be reevaluated.

Sanderson: We have tried to answer that question by depriving eosinophil-producing cultures of IL-5 and then testing whether we could activate the cells. In other words, was this a reversible step as you suggest. Now, when we took away IL-5 from these cells, they both survived and proliferated. What I suspect is happening reflects the micro-environment of these cells, for there is now clear evidence that GM-CSF can bind to the extracellular matrix and be retained in cultures in that way. I think it is possible that IL-5 is doing the same thing, so that we cannot remove this stimulus, which remains on the extracellular matrix, causing the cells to respond over several days. Hence, the question cannot yet be answered.

Wasserman: My question relates to the activity of IgA production in eosinophilia. To see them together would require that the same site on the IL-5 molecule be responsible for both activities. It is a tempting possibilty and it is certainly true for other factors, for which one unique part of the molecule does everything. There appears to be no reason why that must be so and certainly there are no data from human studies to suggest even what part of the IL-5 molecule is active. So couldn't it be possible that there are different cleavage products of IL-5, one of which is important for IgA, one of which is important for eosinophils? Or perhaps the site of production is unique; if IL-5 is made in Peyers patches, that is where you will get IgA.

Sanderson: All these are possibilities but, as I said, there is no good evidence yet.

Gleich: You mentioned that you could measure IL-5 readily, using an ELISA in mouse serum. Can you do so in human serum and do you have any data on human diseases?

Sanderson: No, we don't. Thank you for raising this point. When we use a three-week liquid culture sytem, we can measure eosinophil peroxidase (EPO) production, because neutrophils have disappeared at that point and myeloperoxidase (MPO) does not interfere. In man, myeloperoxidase interferes at all stages; it is not as simple as in the mouse. The assay system for human material is so horrendous we have done very little work trying to detect IL-5 in serum. Until there is a decent assay, that will not happen.

Venge: One of your slides indicated that the granules in the normal cells were atypical. Have you any information of the granuloprotein composition?

Sanderson: No, none whatsoever. We haven't done anything like that yet.

Yukawa: I'm also very interested in the direct interaction between EDF and activation of eosinophils that Professor Vadas mentioned this morning, the priming effect of IL-5, eosinophil superoxide release and ADCC. So could I ask you: is there any possibility that in patients with asthma, that IL-5 has an important role as a priming agent for eosinophil activation? Have you any evidence from patients with asthma?

Sanderson: I do not work with patients. I think it would be unfair for me to attempt to answer that question.

Vadas: The priming situation is seen only in neutrophils; IL-5, GM-CSF and IL-3 provide a direct stimulus of superoxide production in human eosinophils. Eosinophils do not need priming whereas in neutrophils there is no direct effect of these lymphokines, as far as we can detect.

Sanderson: We still don't know if IL-5 is involved in asthma. I think there is absolutely no evidence for that at this stage.

Gleich: Is there an antibody available to IL-5?

Sanderson: We are making them, but we don't have satisfactory monoclonals as yet.

Gleich: I take it, material is not available commercially.

Sanderson: Not available to me!

Kay: Do you know anything about the active site?

Sanderson: No, nothing is known about the active site.

Kay: And, you haven't got a radioimmunoassay? Presumably without one, questions of the role of IL-5 for instance in Christopher's hypereosinophilic syndromes, would be rather difficult to ask because of GM-CSF and IL-3.

Sanderson: Yes, but it won't be very long before we can start asking those questions.

Gleich: There is one question I have. You mentioned that, in the mouse, you can utilize the peroxidase assay to detect eosinophils because there is relatively little MPO in the mouse neutrophil. In human it's rather the opposite. There is quite a bit of MPO in the human neutrophil. It is my understanding that the cyanide-resistant peroxidase assay only applies to fixed cells on a slide, and doesn't work with cell supernatants. Is that your understanding? Or can anyone else comment on that?

Sanderson: I can say that we have tried very hard using various inhibitors to make an assay that is specific for either MPO or EPO. We are unable to achieve the sort of precision you need for these sort of assays. That is all that I can say. You cannot simply add MPO inhibitor and then detect EPO, and say that you are measuring eosinophils; it is not clean enough.

Gleich: But are you referring to analysis of fluid EPO and MPO, or are you referring to activities on cells that have been put down on a glass slide?

Sanderson: The assay is done in the presence of triton to lyse the cells. There is immediate release of peroxidase which is then assayed in solution.

Spry: I've always been worried that we are not assaying *in vitro* what is happening *in vivo*, in the sense that if you give a eosinopoietic stimulus to a normal individual you can induce accelerated production of eosinophils within 24 hours and this peaks at about 3 or 4 days, so that you have massive numbers of cells transferred into the blood within 2 days and certainly peaking at 4 days. Now, none of the *in vitro* systems seem to come close to this in their capacity to induce an eosinophil response. I wonder, therefore, what you think about the assay systems as they stand at the moment. Don't you think that we are perhaps limiting them in that we are not adding to them some accessory components, perhaps multiple factors that are required to reproduce the *in vivo* events which are really quite different. I think that your system or the agar system are very slow, giving very small effects. Perhaps we should not be too excited about these molecules as eosinopoietic components, as there may be other factors and other systems which are obviously going to accelerate this phenomenon. These could be endothelial cells or the nerve cells in the bone marrow so that perhaps we haven't got the full story. I'd be interested in your views on this dichotomy.

Sanderson: In the mouse, the system is clearer. There is a much closer correlation between the production of IL-5, its appearance in the serum and the production of eosinophils. In the human systems, I agree with you, that the rate of differentiation *in vitro* is very, very slow and it is difficult to imagine how bone marrow can pour out so many eosinophils so quickly if it takes 14 days before you see a single eosinophil *in vitro*. So, there is no correlation between *in vitro* and *in vivo* rates. I'm not sure that this problem relates to factors. I think the micro-environment is probably the critical factor in these experiments. That is why in the mouse we can get beautiful eosinophil differentiation in the liquid cultures, but very poor results in agar. It's not quite as clear cut in human cultures. It is probable that in the bottom of a little well you have the micro-environment that you need, allowing the cell–cell interactions to take place; but you are right, we are really only scratching the surface of what is going on in the bone marrow.

Spry: It seems to me that you are providing so much growth factor in these studies, that you really excluded a role for accessory factors in the story. I mean, you can't imagine these sort of concentrations being produced in a bone marrow environment, or perhaps you do.

Sanderson: Oh yes, if you work back from the levels we can detect in the serum of a mouse, and you remember that the turnover of the growth factors is enormously rapid and they are bound in the bone marrow by the specific receptor and possibly by the glycocalyx of other cells, then I think you will have very high concentrations locally.

Kay: But, Colin surely you have some data which you presented previously on pre-culturing with IL-3 and then IL-5.

Sanderson: Yes, now that we have recombinant IL-3, we are repeating these experiments in both mouse and man. The results are a little bit controversial and we have not really got good data yet but, in our preliminary experiments, IL-1 (haemopoietin 1) is actually a very poor inducer of the eosinophil. IL-3 works a dream but IL-1 we find is almost irrelevant in these systems. There are factors involved in these early stages but really the crunch will come when we put the IL-5 back into a mouse, to determine if it does induce eosinophilia. And that's really the important experiment which we haven't done yet.

Kay: But, is it the IL-3 which is promoting the stem cell to the eosinophil progenitor stage?

Sanderson: That's what it looks like and it fits in with the dogma about IL-3 but we have no evidence yet.

Vadas: My question was very much related to this theme. I've just heard the news of the monkey trials in which treatment of IL-3 was followed by GM-CSF. Essentially, IL-3 allows a subthreshold dose of GM-CSF to work like a dream. So it looks as if IL-3 pre-sets the bone marrow responsiveness to GM-CSF. The question with IL-3 is, do you find that the bone marrow also responds to GM-CSF a lot better? Does IL-3 pre-set the bone marrow to all the other cytokines?

Sanderson: Yes, IL-3 seems to work in this way. It seems to prime the bone marrow to respond to GM-CSF.

Vadas: OK, then from the parasitized mice, you have a bone marrow that seems to be leading to eosinophilopoiesis and not leading to neutrophilopoiesis. Is that correct?

Sanderson: No, that is not quite correct. A parasitized mouse is a complex beast and there are an increased number of all the haemopoietic lineages including the erythroid lineages. One point I should make, which is important for the earlier discussions, is that in these mice the major haemopoietic organ becomes the spleen. Haemopoiesis starts in the bone marrow, but within a few days the spleen size is increased three or four times and progresses to eight times its original size. The number of eosinophils produced in the spleen are 20 times greater than those produced in the bone marrow. Haemopoiesis occurring in the spleen is identified by visible mitosis and immature forms. Furthermore, around the granuloma in the liver caused by this parasite, you can also see immature forms and mitosis. There is no doubt that, in the mouse, eosinophil haemopoiesis can take place at sites other than the bone marrow.

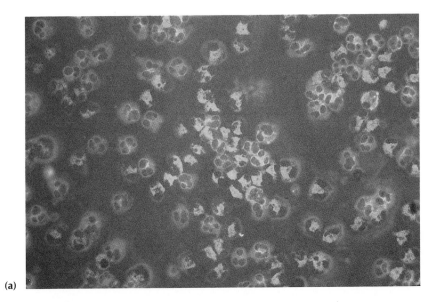

(a)

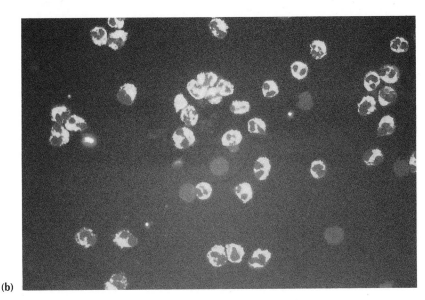

(b)

Plate I. Surface IgA on human eosinophils. Cytocentrifuged preparations of granulocyte suspensions from a filariasis infected patient were made and fixed with methanol. Unlabelled anti-human IgA was (a) added or (b) omitted. Slides were further stained with chromotrope 2R in order to identify eosinophils appearing in red. Fluorescein labelled anti-goat antiserum was then added.

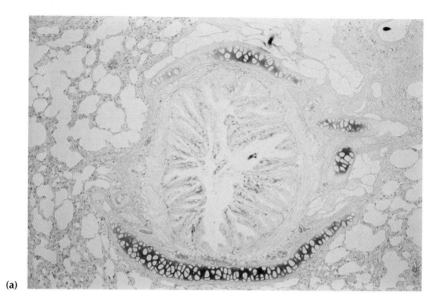

(a)

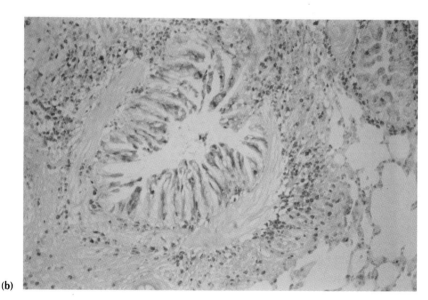

(b)

Plate II. Histopathology of the lungs stained by Giemsa stain (x200): (a) control guinea pig before exposure to antigen; (b) control guinea pig at 6 h; (c) control guinea pig at 24 h; (d) guinea-pig pretreated by AH21–132 before exposure to antigen; (e) guinea-pig pretreated by AH21–132 at 6 h; (f) guinea-pig pretreated by AH21–132 at 24 h.

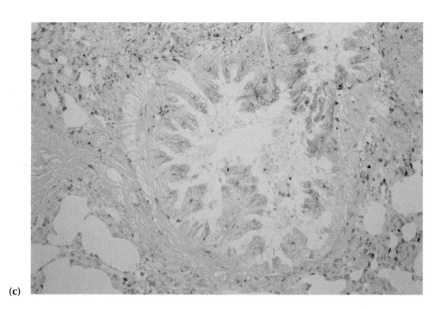

(c)

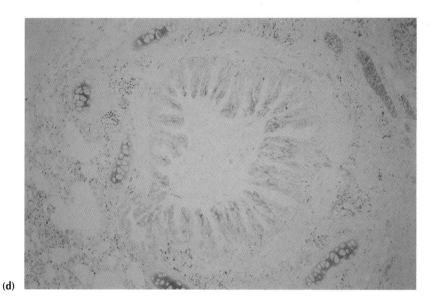

(d)

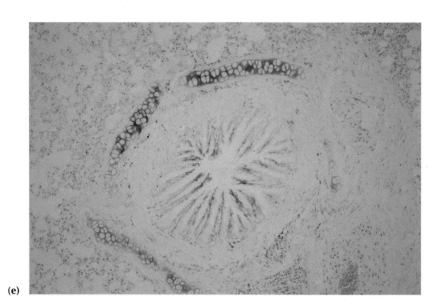

(e)

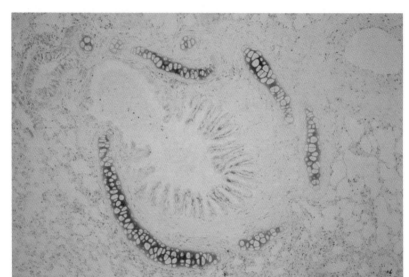

(f)

4

Immunoglobulin-mediated Activation of Eosinophils

M. Capron, C. Leprevost, L. Prin, M. Tomassini, G. Torpier, S. MacDonald* and A. Capron

Centre d'Immunologie et de Biologie Parasitaire, Unité Mixte INSERM U167-CNRS 624 Institut Pasteur de Lille, France

* The Johns Hopkins University of Medicine, Clinical Immunology Division, Baltimore, Md, USA

4.1 INTRODUCTION

Allergic manifestations represent an important component of morbidity in human populations. Since the discovery in the last 20 years of the cellular and humoral mechanisms underlying immediate hypersensitivity reactions, one main concept has largely dominated the field of allergy and strongly influenced the general approaches of prevention and therapy. This general concept is related to the major role played by chemical mediators of cellular origin, in the network of events leading to clinical manifestations of allergic reactions such as asthma. In this respect, both at the experimental and

Eosinophils in Asthma
ISBN 0-12-506452-7

applied research levels, exclusive attention has been paid to mast cell and basophil derived mediators and to molecules able to control mediator release under IgE-dependent triggering.

An entirely novel approach, developed in our laboratory during the last ten years and now widely confirmed, has allowed to be demonstrated that this concept based on the intervention of an unique cell population was not exclusive (1). In a broad sense, allergic reactions are the results of a cell interaction network involving the release of pharmacological mediators by other cells than the classical mast cells or basophils. In this context, our initial discovery of the existence of IgE receptors on eosinophils has drawn the attention on their direct participation, so far underestimated, in the basic mechanisms of hypersensitivity reactions (2).

Eosinophils are incriminated in the pathology of asthma by releasing various newly and preformed mediators among which specific components such as the granule cationic proteins (major basic protein, MBP; eosinophil cationic protein, ECP; eosinophil peroxidase, EPO) directly involved in tissue damage (reviewed in ref. 3). However, very few studies have concerned the precise mechanisms of mediator release. During our initial studies in parasitic diseases, we showed that eosinophils were able to interact specifically with restricted isotypes of immunoglobulins (4). In the present work we have investigated the release of eosinophil granule proteins in response to various immunological stimuli, such as IgE, IgG or soluble IgE-binding factors. These findings associated with results obtained by using electron microscopy and immunogold staining with the various antibodies directed against the granule proteins, allowed us to suggest a selectivity in the mediators released by eosinophils.

In addition, we report preliminary results concerning the existence and the functional role of a receptor for IgA on eosinophils, leading to the concept of a particular interaction of eosinophils with immunoglobulins present in the tissues and their participation to local immune responses.

4.2   EOSINOPHILS AND IgE IMMUNOGLOBULINS

4.2.1   IgE Receptors

IgE receptors have been clearly demonstrated on human eosinophils and they participate directly in the effector function of eosinophils against parasite larvae (1, 5). The parallel inhibition of IgE receptors of eosinophils, macrophages and platelets, by a polyclonal antiserum directed against IgE receptors of a B cell line, indicated that these IgE-Fc receptors (FcεR) are antigenically related (1). The production of a monoclonal antibody (BB10) raised against human FcεR-positive eosinophils and able to inhibit the IgE-dependent cytotoxicity of eosinophils, platelets and monocytes, has confirmed the common antigenicity of these FcεR, now referred to as FcεRII (1, 6).

A common feature of these FcεRII is their increased expression on activated cells. In the particular situation of human eosinophils, IgE-dependent effector function seemed to be restricted to a subpopulation of eosinophils with low density (hypodense), suggesting that the presence of a functional FcεR could be considered as one marker of eosinophil heterogeneity (5). This hypothesis was confirmed by using the monoclonal antibody (mAb) BB10, produced by immunization of mice with hypodense blood and lung eosinophils. This mAb directed against FcεRII was able selectively to stain hypodense and not normodense eosinophils, by immunofluorescence (6).

In addition, this mAb allowed us to characterize biochemically the eosinophil receptor for IgE. The specific binding of radioiodinated BB10, reduced into a monomeric form, was measured by using the Scatchard analysis: a mean number of 10^5 binding sites per cell and an association constant (K_a) of 10^7 M^{-1} was calculated for hypodense eosinophils. Analysis of the molecules constitutive of eosinophil FcεR was performed by using immunosorbent chromatography of eosinophil detergent extracts, passed over either IgE or BB10 immunosorbents. Under reducing conditions, 3 polypeptide fragments were obtained with apparent molecular weights of 45–50, 23 and 15 kDa (the latter being more prominent in the case of the BB10 immunosorbent). The similarities between the SDS-PAGE patterns of eosinophil extracts eluted from IgE and from BB10 immunosorbent confirmed the specificity of BB10 for the IgE receptor. Finally, comparative analysis suggested that the FcεRII of human eosinophils and of a human macrophage cell line (U937) are structurally related, and differ from the high affinity FcεRI present on basophils and mast cells (7).

The demonstration of surface IgE on eosinophils from patients with increased IgE levels, and particularly on lung eosinophils, confirmed the biological relevance of the interaction between eosinophils and IgE antibodies (8). In order to investigate the role of these cytophilic IgE in eosinophil function and to evaluate their specificity, further experiments measuring the release of various mediators were then performed.

4.2.2 Selective Release of Mediators

Surface IgE-bearing eosinophils were purified from hypereosinophilic patients and incubated with anti-IgE, anti-IgG or with medium. EPO was measured in the supernatants by a method based on chemiluminescence (9). Incubation of eosinophils with anti-IgE antibodies but not with anti-IgG induced exocytosis of EPO. The comparison between "hypodense" and "normodense" eosinophil populations confirmed our previous results on the functional heterogeneity of human eosinophils: both populations bound IgE but only the hypodense eosinophils were able to degranulate in response to an IgE stimulus. To demonstrate the antibody specificity of these cytophilic IgE, EPO was measured in the supernatants after incubation of eosinophils with various antigens. Only the antigens related to the patient infection and none of the unrelated antigens induced extracellular release of EPO. The fact that EPO was released by a secretory process and not as the consequence of cell death was shown by the kinetic experiments of EPO versus LDH (Lactate dehydrogenase, a cytoplasmic enzyme): EPO release was detectable as soon as 15 min after addition of the stimulus, and reached a plateau at 1 h, whereas no LDH could be detected in the same supernatants.

Since these results have been mainly obtained from patients with parasitic infections (9), we have performed similar studies with allergic patients. Eosinophils were purified from such patients exhibiting relatively low percentages of blood eosinophils. They were incubated for 1 h with various doses of allergen or anti-IgE. The determination of eosinophil peroxidase (EPO) in the supernatants was carried out as above by using chemiluminescence (CL). For the homogenization of individual results, they were expressed as the index of EPO release, after subtraction of the controls without cells according to the formula:

$$\text{EPO index:}\ \frac{\underset{\text{(Eos + stimulus)}}{\text{CL units}} - \underset{\text{(stimulus without Eos)}}{\text{CL units}}}{\underset{\text{(Eos + medium)}}{\text{CL units}}}$$

As shown in Figure 1, summarizing the results of 6 allergic patients and 13 non-allergic patients, significant levels of EPO (2–12 times more than in the controls) could be detected in the supernatants. Only allergens related to the patient allergy and giving positivity in the skin tests induced extracellular release of EPO. However, no release of EPO was obtained when the same allergens were added to eosinophils from non-allergic patients. The participation of IgE antibodies in this mechanism was suggested by the very significant correlation between the index of EPO release after incubation with allergen or with anti-IgE ($r = 0.93$; $p < 0.001$). The interference of a spontaneous chemiluminescence reaction due to the presence of superoxide anions and in-

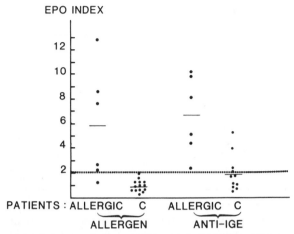

Fig. 1   EPO release in allergic patients. Purified eosinophils from allergic or non-allergic patients were incubated either with the specific allergen or with anti-IgE at the optimal concentration. After 1 h incubation at 37°C, cells were centrifuged and EPO was measured in the supernatants by chemiluminescence. The results were expressed as EPO index (an index superior to 2 was considered as significant).

dependent of peroxidase was ruled out by the fact that EPO was measured after an overnight stay of the centrifugation supernatants at $+4°C$. In contrast, the spontaneous chemiluminescence reaction requires the presence of cells and must be performed very rapidly after activation since these oxygen metabolites are very labile. It would be certainly very interesting to perform a radioimmunoassay using specific antibodies directed against EPO in order to confirm the presence of the EPO molecule in these supernatants. However, the enzymatic assay has the advantage of measuring the molecule under a biologically active form, which is not the case for a radioimmunoassay.

These results suggested that cell-bound IgE with very restricted antibody specificity could play a role in the activation of hypodense eosinophils in inducing the release of a granule protein with potent cytolytic functions. Since we have demonstrated that surface IgE molecules were present particularly on tissue eosinophils from patients with lung diseases (8), we can extrapolate that such a mediator released as a consequence of interactions between IgE and eosinophils might participate in pathology, both directly since EPO was shown to be involved in cytolytic processes against lung cells and indirectly since EPO supplemented with H_2O_2 and halide is able to induce mast cell degranulation.

Using the same conditions of activation as for EPO release, the exocytosis of other granule components, namely MBP, ECP and EDN was measured by

Table 1   Comparison between release of MBP, ECP and EDN (RIA using *polyclonal* antibodies)

Incubation of human eosinophils 60 min at 37°C with	MBP ng/ml	% of total	ECP ng/ml	% of total	EDN ng/ml	% of total
Medium	<22	–	55±25	2±0.9	303±49	4±0.6
Specific Ag	262±4	65	325±119	11±4	833±300	10±1.6
Unrelated Ag	<22	–	123±64	5±3	283±57	4±1
Anti-IgE	55±29	11±7	142±71	5±1	397±78	5±0.7
Anti-IgG	<22	–	139±4	3.8±1	343±108	4±0.5
TRITON	487±60		3642±1296		7375±1453	

using radioimmunoassays with the corresponding polyclonal antibodies. These assays were performed in Dr Gerald Gleich's laboratory in Rochester (Minnesota, USA).

As shown in Table 1, the three cationic proteins were released after addition of the specific antigens, confirming the antibody specificity of cytophilic immunoglobulins. However, the participation of IgE was not clearly demonstrated except for MBP release. These results suggested that, as expected, EPO was not the only mediator released after IgE dependent activation, but that a major granule component with cytolytic activities for a large variety of target cells (MBP) was also released.

In collaboration with Dr Pochun Tai and Professor Christopher Spry (St George's Medical School, London) we evaluated in the same supernatants, the levels of Eosinophil Cationic Protein (ECP) by a radioimmunoassay using antiECP monoclonal antibodies. As shown in Figure 2, which represents the mean of several experiments, ECP was not detected after incubation of eosinophils with antigen or with anti-IgE, but was very strikingly detected after addition of anti-IgG. These results showing no correlation between EPO and ECP release suggested a variability in the response of eosinophils to different stimuli (IgE v. IgG). Not only the mediators released after IgE versus IgG dependent activation were different but the kinetics of release was also different. IgE-dependent activation induced EPO release with a peak at 1 h whereas IgG-dependent activation induced ECP release with a peak at 4 h.

These results were recently confirmed by studies on a factor named HRF (histamine releasing factor), described by Dr L. Lichtenstein's group at the Johns Hopkins University (Baltimore) as able to induce histamine release after addition to IgE-bearing basophils (10). When surface IgE-bearing eosinophils were incubated with this semi-purified HRF factor, EPO was

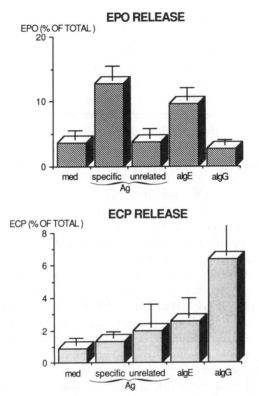

Fig. 2 Differential release of EPO and ECP by eosinophils. Purified eosinophils were incubaed with various stimuli (specific or unrelated antigens, anti-human IgE or anti-human IgG antibodies) for 1 h at 37°C. EPO levels in the supernatants were expressed as the percentage of the total release obtained after cell lysis with Triton × 100.

detected in the supernatants but, as similar to the IgE dependent activation, not ECP. Moreover, studies performed on 10 different patients showed a highly significant correlation between the levels of EPO release (measured in CL units) after addition of HRF or anti-IgE ($r = 0.96$, $p < 0.001$), suggesting the participation of surface IgE antibodies in both cases.

These results confirmed our hypothesis of a selectivity in the mediators released by IgE or IgG dependent activation of human eosinophils, and raised several questions, including: how could two molecules (EPO and ECP), present in the same compartment of eosinophil granules, be separately released, if eosinophils degranulate by a mechanism of granule exocytosis like for the mast cells? Electron microscopy technology was therefore used to investigate this mechanism of mediator release. During the time of incubation of eosinophils with the stimulus (30–60 min), very few granules seemed exocytosed as a whole. In contrast, it was possible to see pictures of fusion of adjacent granules, formation of buds and vesicles at the level of the granule membrane, and presence of (secretory?) channels between the granules and the plasmatic membrane. The release of mediators would therefore be due to a secretion of some (but not all) granule components from the granules towards the exterior.

This attractive hypothesis was investigated *in vivo* in the case of a patient with eosinophilic gastroenteritis. Electron microscopy studies of perendoscopic biopsies obtained from the descending duodenum showed eosinophils presenting simultaneously the various features of activation and especially the inversion of the electron density of the crystalloid. Vesicles were formed at the level of the crystalloid, which led to a loss of material from the granule, as shown by the changes in electron density.

We also used the colloidal gold procedure, by incubating the same tissue sections with monospecific polyclonal antibodies directed against MBP (kindly donated by Dr Gleich) or against EPO (kindly donated by Dr Venge, Uppsala, Sweden), or with monoclonal anti-ECP antibodies (EG2, kindly provided by Dr Tai in London). The binding of these antibodies was revealed by using colloidal gold grains coated with appropriate reagent (anti-rabbit or anti-mouse Ig respectively). This technology allowed us to confirm, in resting eosinophils, the presence of MBP at the crystalloid level and EPO and ECP in the matrix. By using this technology it was possible to identify in activated eosinophils the loss of MBP outside of the granule corresponding to the inversion of the density, whereas EPO and ECP were normally distributed in the granule matrix (11).

The *in vivo* studies confirmed that our findings concerning the selectivity of mediators released by eosinophils were not an *in vitro* artefact and that all the steps of eosinophil "degranulation" could probably be observed, from the very discrete secretion of mediators, until cell lysis. Similar experiments are now in progress in order to follow the kinetics of the release of various mediators after *in vitro* activation.

This new concept of "selectivity of mediators released by eosinophils" might have some implications in pathology and specially in allergy.

Three main factors would therefore influence release of mediators by eosinophils:

1. the stimulus of activation (IgE v. IgG): the mediators released in diseases associated with increased IgE levels such as allergic states, or not, like in

the hypereosinophilic syndrome (HES) might be different, or their relative importance might be different;
2. the kinetics of the response: different mediators could participate in the immediate versus the late phase of the asthmatic reaction; our results showing a peak of ECP at 4 h are consistent with the presence of higher levels of ECP in the bronchoalveolar lavages during the late phase reaction;
3. the eosinophil heterogeneity: the IgE-dependent release of mediators requires a functional FcεR, only present on some eosinophil subpopulations. The ratio of FcεR positive versus negative eosinophils might vary according to the different tissues or organs; therefore, the mediators released in a given localization might differ.

4.2.3 IgE Binding Factors

The above results showed that the release of eosinophil mediators can be induced not only by antigens or anti-IgE but also by soluble factors such as HRF. HRF, which is present in nasal lavage fluids and blister fluids during the late cutaneous reaction, has a MW of 15–30 kDa, and can be considered in some aspects as an "IgE binding factor". It is produced *in vitro* by lung macrophages and platelets, both cell populations bearing in common the second receptor for IgE (FcεRII) (10). However no similar studies have been related with the production of such IgE binding factors by eosinophils.

In the first series of experiments, purified human eosinophils were metabolically labelled with ^{35}S-Met and incubated in MEM lacking Met in the presence of FMLP as a stimulatory agent. After an overnight incubation at 37°C, cells were centrifuged and the supernatants were submitted to immunoprecipitation by the mAb anti-FcεRII BB10 or by a control IgM. SDS-Page analysis followed by autoradiography of the molecules immunoprecipitated revealed a major band at 15 kDa, recognized by BB10 only and not by the control IgM. The further step was to investigate whether such soluble factors, synthetized by eosinophils and released in the supernatants, were able to bind IgE. Similar culture supernatants of unlabelled eosinophils were submitted to western blotting procedure under reduced conditions. Two major bands were detected at 15 and 18 kDa, both able to bind the mAb anti-FcεRII and IgE. These findings indicate that FcεR + hypodense eosinophils are able to release soluble factors of a molecular weight comparable to the previously described IgE binding factors, and able to bind IgE. The functional aspects of eosinophil IgE BF are presently under investigation.

4.3   EOSINOPHILS AND IgA IMMUNOGLOBULINS

4.3.1   Surface IgA

During the course of our studies on the presence of surface IgE on eosinophils from hypereosinophilic patients, we have investigated the presence of other immunoglobulin isotypes. Granulocyte suspensions from patients with filariasis infections were coated on slides by cytocentrifugation. After fixation with methanol, they were incubated with various anti-immunoglobulin antisera and further incubated with a second antibody labelled with fluorescein. Very strikingly, whereas the presence of surface IgE was not easily detected by this insensitive technology, clearcut fluorescence of eosinophil membrane was observed after addition of fluorescein labelled human anti-IgA antibodies (Plate I). This positive result was only obtained in the case of eosinophils from filariasis patients and not in the uninfected controls. As expected, the contaminating neutrophils were also strongly positive. These findings associated to similar results obtained in the case of intestinal eosinophils from mice infected with an intestinal cestode parasite *Hymenolepis diminuta* (12), suggested the existence of IgA receptors on eosinophils.

4.3.2   Receptors for IgA

To further investigate this hypothesis, we measured the binding of monomeric IgA to purified human eosinophils (> 95% purity), by flow cytofluorometry analysis after staining with fluorescein-labelled anti-human IgA. Between 5 and 40% of eosinophils were able to bind IgA, Moreover, the proportion of surface IgA bearing eosinophils increased in the case of allergic patients. These results confirmed our initial studies on eosinophils fixed onto slides and very interestingly showed similarities between the percentages of eosinophils able to bind IgE and IgA (8). The association between the two receptors at the level of individual cells is presently under investigation. More recently, experiments of binding of radiolabelled seric IgA were performed and showed the existence of a saturable binding site for IgA not only on blood but also on tissue eosinophils.

4.3.3   Functional Aspects of IgA Receptors

To know whether the IgA receptors could be associated with eosinophil activation we evaluated the comparative release of EPO either after addition of anti-IgE or of anti-IgA. A significant release of EPO (between 2.5 and 6 times more than in controls) was obtained after addition of anti-IgA. These results suggested that, similarly to IgE, surface IgA could participate in eosinophil activation, by inducing the release of mediators.

4.4 CONCLUSION

In addition to several studies reporting the role of eosinophils in bronchial asthma (numbers of eosinophils increased in the bronchoalveolar lavage fluids or presence of specific eosinophil meditors in the lavages or in tissue sections), our results showed that eosinophils, through their surface immunoglobulins, were able to interact with antigens, and to release their various mediators. Among the various immunoglobulin isotypes, surface IgE and IgA seemed particularly involved in mediator release and these findings might have *in vivo* implications in the context of tissue reactions, especially in the lungs and in the intestine.

In addition, our results suggest a differential release of the various granule mediators, as also recently demonstrated in the case of release of ECP and EPX in response to activation by opsonized zymosan (see Ch. 10 this volume). Moreover, electron microscopy studies indicate that mediator release was not due to exocytosis of the whole granules but rather to a secretory process from the granules to the exterior. This selectivity in mediator release might depend upon the conditions of eosinophil activation and might also vary according to the target organs.

Finally, the third message is related to soluble IgE binding factors, such as HRF, which is able to induce mediator release by various cell populations (basophils, eosinophils and also platelets). These factors, probably released by FcεRII-bearing cells, are present in the biological fluids *in vivo*, and it's possible to speculate that they might activate surface IgE-bearing cells, in the absence of antigens, and therefore be involved in chronic diseases.

Kinetic studies of eosinophil activation via immunoglobulins would be of interest in order clearly to establish the role of eosinophils both in the early and in the late phase of asthmatic reaction.

REFERENCES

1. Capron, A., Dessaint, J. P., Capron, M., Joseph, M., Ameisen, J. C. and Tonnel, A. B. (1986). *Immunology Today* 7, 15–18.

2. Capron, M., Capron, A., Dessaint, J. P., Torpier, G., Johansson, S. G. O. and Prin, L. (1981). *J. Immunol*, **126**, 2087–2092.
3. Gleich, G. J. and Adolphson, C. R. (1986). *Adv. Immunol.* **39**, 177–253.
4. Capron, A., Dessaint, J. P., Haque, A. and Capron, M. (1982). *Progr. Allergy* **31**, 234–267.
5. Capron, M., Spiegelberg, H. L., Prin, L., Bennich, H., Butterworth, A. E., Pierce, R. J., Ouaissi, M. A. and Capron, A. (1984). *J. Immunol.* **232**, 462–468.
6. Capron, M., Jouault, T., Prin, L., Joseph, M., Ameisen, J. C., Butterworth, A. E., Papin, J. P., Kusnierz, J. P. and Capron, A. (1986). *J. Exp. Med.* **164**, 72–89.
7. Jouault, T., Capron, M., Balloul, J. M., Ameisen, J. C. and Capron, A. (1988). *Eur. J. Immunol.* **18**, 237–241.
8. Capron, M., Kusnierz, J. P., Prin, L., Spiegelberg, H. L., Ovlaque, G., Gosset, P., Tonnel, A. B. and Capron, A. (1985). *J. Immunol* **134**, 3013–3018.
9. Khalife, J., Capron, M., Cesbron, J. Y., Tai, P. C.,Taelman, H., Prin, L. and Capron, A. (1986). *J. Immunol* **137**, 1659–1664.
10. Liu, M. C., Proud, D., Lichtenstein, L. M., MacGlashan, D. W. Jr., Schleimer, R. P., Adkinson, N. F. Jr., Kagey-Sobotka, A., Schulman, E. S. and Plaut, M. (1986). *J. Immunol.* **136**, 2588–2595.
11. Torpier, G., Colombel, J. F., Mathieu-Chandelier, C., Dessaint, J. P., Cortot, A., Paris, J. C. and Capron, M. (1988). *Clin. Exp. Immunol.* **74**, 404–408.
12. Vandervorst, E., Dhont, H., Cesbron, J. Y., Capron, M., Dessaint, J. P. and Capron, A. (1988). *Int. Arch. All. Appl. Immunol.* **87**, 281–285.

DISCUSSION

Makino (Chairman): Is there a difference between numbers of IgA receptors on hypodense and normodense cells?

Capron: We have not yet looked at the difference between the hypodense and normodense cells, but we need to perform these experiments and we need also to perform double labelling experiments to know whether IgE and IgA are detected on the same eosinophil populations. I have no answer for the moment.

Kay: I think there are at least two papers on IgA receptors on neutrophils. I know Peter Henson's group back in the seventies, showed that labelled monomeric IgA bound to neutrophils. I wondered if you could comment on that in view of your findings.

Capron: Yes, we wished to compare neutrophils and eosinophils, so we searched the literature for the molecular weight, the affinity of IgA receptor on neutrophils and the average number of receptors on neutrophils. I was very surprised to find that very few papers contain this kind of information. This is surprising because neutrophils are easy to purify and neutrophil receptors probably have higher affinity for IgAs than the eosinophil receptor. So, now we have started experiments on neutrophils exactly like those we performed on eosinophils comparing the binding of monomeric and secretory IgA with radiolabelled IgA using Scatchard analysis. These experiments should answer all the questions.

Kay: Could I also ask you about the chemoluminescence assay. I'm a little confused about this because I would expect that an eosinophil, which has been activated and has undergone partial reduction, with the formation of partial reduction products, to react in a chemoluminescence assay and I wonder how you distinguish these products from your EPO.

Capron: Possibly Lionel Prin could answer that question better than I can. The levels of spontaneous chemoluminescence are very different in the presence and absence of hydrogen peroxide (H_2O_2). So we compare the chemoluminescence under both conditions and we also standardize measurements using a given quantity of horse radish peroxidase as a standard.

Prin: When we studied eosinophil activation by phorbol myristate acetate (PMA), we observed that hypodense cells showed a very low response to PMA, because it seems these cells are activated *in vivo*. The activation of hypodense cells with a specific activator, immunoglobulins or lymphokines, caused a quite different response, as detected by the EPO and chemoluminescence assay. The responses of normodense or hypodense cells to non-specific stimuli are quite different. It's difficult to compare the peroxidase assay and the chemoluminescence assay, because chemoluminescence reflects all oxidative metabolism. However, the sensitivities of hypodense and normodense cells to specific or non-specific activators are quite different. Hypodense cells reveal *in vivo* activation or priming so that when we activate these cells with a second signal (immunoglobulins or lymphokines), we can easily activate the cells. However, when we study normodense cells from normal persons, the level of activation is quite different; normodense cells are very difficult to activate.

Capron: I would like to add that the levels of spontaneous chemoluminescence by hypodense cells are very low in the absence of the stimulus anti-Ig. When we started to use this chemoluminescence assay for the measurement of peroxidase, we used rat eosinophils and compared the enzymatic assay with the chemoluminescence assay and we could show a good correlation. We had a good correlation but the chemoluminescence assay is much more sensitive than the enzymatic assay. To answer precisely your question, I think that the presence of reduction products different from EPO can be ruled out by the fact that the chemiluminescence reaction to evaluation EPO was performed on cell-free supernatants kept overnight at $+4°C$. In these conditions the various oxygen metabolites eventually produced, which are very labile, can be hardly detected.

Gleich: Is the release by histamine releasing factor of EPO in your chemoluminescence assay confined to the hypodense subset or the normodense subset or both?

Capron: The problem of comparing hypodense and normodense eosinophils is that it is very difficult to obtain normodense eosinophils. When we use this chemoluminescence assay, we need 5×10^6 eosinophils per millilitre, so we mainly perform our experiments with hypodense eosinophils. To answer your question, we have not compared normodense and hypodense eosinophils. We have only compared the reaction of hypodense eosinophils to anti-IgE stimulus versus HRF stimulus. We have not looked at normodense eosinophils.

Vadas: A couple of points which require clarification. First of all, does the ECP release need protein synthesis?

Capron: Nobody has looked to this point, I think!

Vadas: The second question is, you said that ECP is released by anti-IgG.

Capron: Yes.

Vadas: But, in the schistosomula assay, where you find ECP, it is IgE.

Capron: That is a good point; it is a paradox. When we performed our experiments, comparing the levels of ECP measured by the polyclonal antibodies of Dr Gleich and the levels of ECP measured by the monoclonal antibodies, we observed intriguing differences. These experiments have been done using cells from filariasis patients only, because they have many more eosinophils and more IgE antibodies. When we looked at the presence of proteins on the schistosomula, we are very surprised because we expected to see EPO or MBP but the only molecule present at the interface was ECP detected by the polyclonal antibodies. I would like to ask Dr Gleich and Dr Spry, what is the difference between the molecules seen by the polyclonal anti-ECP and not seen by the two different monoclonal antibodies? Can you answer that question?

Gleich: Well, ECP is extremely polymorphic and the polymorphisms are probably due to carbohydrate additions since endo F and endo H, I think it was endo F, take the molecule back to about a 16 kd monomer form. So I suppose it's conceivable that the monoclonal might be recognizing an antigenic determinant, recognizing one of these subspecies, which could indeed be preferentially reduced. I don't see any argument against that hypothesis; on the other hand I'm not sure that I would believe it.

Capron: Have you performed cross-inhibition experiments between the monoclonal antibodies and the polyclonals?

Gleich: No.

Vadas: You have apparently the same band identified by IgE and BB10. Now, can you pre-clear with one of them?

Capron: We have not performed those experiments. It's a good idea. To check the specificity of the reagents BB10, IgE and anti-IgM and anti-IgE, we used two different clones of U937. One clone is able to bind BB10 and IgE and the second one is able to bind only BB10 and not IgE in the fluorescence assay. We have a clear result with the clone which binds both BB10 and IgE, in the supernatants we can detect both bands, and with the clone which binds only BB10 by fluorescence we detect in the supernatants one band which is recognized by BB10 and not by IgE. The controls using anti-IgE and anti-IgM are negative.

Vadas: One more question. I hope you'll forgive me for this. You probably will be a bit angry but I think the finding is so important of this selective degranulation that I'm going to say that I don't believe the electron microscope evidence that you showed. Have you checked using morphometry, counting a hundred grains in a cell. Actually, each example looks pretty good, but it's such an important thing that it would be nice to back it up quantitatively.

Capron: As I told you, it is an hypothesis. In the literature there are very few papers concerning the mechanisms of the release of mediators. I propose the hypothesis that some molecules can be released in some situations, whereas others are not released. I think everybody now can work on that question.

Vadas: Yes, it is a terribly important concept.

Gleich: The first comment relates to the morphologic differences between normodense and hypodense cells. There are several manuscripts in the literature, one of which is in press by Dr Fukuda and Dr Peters from our laboratory and in that study it was found that the quantities of eosinophil granule proteins per 10^6 hypodense cells were considerably less than in 10^6 normodense cells, but the numbers of granules were the same. The granules by morphometry appeared to be smaller, which is an interesting difference. My second comment relates to your finding of the reversal of staining. Ann

Dvorak will be pleased as she speculated some time ago that the reversal of staining would be due to loss of MBP. MBP is a powerful cytotoxin, which will kill tumor cells within 15 minutes and maybe within a shorter period of time. What consequences do you think that would have for the cell? Do you have any explanation for this selective loss?

Capron: In the case of the schistosomula assay, the killing assay, we looked only after 1 h contact between the target parasites, antibodies and eosinophils. After 1 h we noticed only ECP in the deposit. That does not mean that investigation at other times might not detect a different composition of the deposits. I don't say that only ECP can kill the parasites, because it has been shown that other molecules, MBP for instance, are involved in the case of IgG-dependent killing. Nobody has carefully looked at the IgE-dependent assay. It is likely that various molecules can be cytotoxic for the parasite target, but after 1 h we have only seen ECP in this particular experiment. It is only one experiment.

Gleich: Dr Parker in our laboratory showed rather convincingly that MBP is quite cytotoxic for the micro-filaria of *Brugia pahangi* and *Brugia malayii*.

Townley: Yes, I would like to clarify the difference between hypodense eosinophils and normodense in terms of IgE receptors. Do you have any quantitative comparisons? Secondly, in your studies with HRF in collaboration with Susan MacDonald, you used several HRF factors, derived from platelets, nasal mucus, and I believe macrophages; do they all activate the eosinophils equally and release EPO and express IgE receptors?

Capron: The first question about the IgE receptors on hypodense and normodense eosinophils. Using the Scatchard analysis and the binding of radiolabelled IgE, we could only detect binding of sufficient affinity on intermediate density and hypodense cells. So, we suggest that receptors on normodense have low affinity and cannot be detected by this technology. In respect of difference between degranulation in response to anti-IgE for hypodense versus normodense, we were very surprised to see that surface IgE can be detected both on normodense and hypodense cells. The difference is the response to the activation signal. So you have IgE bound to both types of cell, but only hypodense cells are able to respond to anti-IgE by degranulation and by releasing factors. To answer your second question, we have only used HRF, semi-purified from nasal fluids

Gleich: That is an interesting point which I think Dr Kay might like to comment on. Because, I think, he found IgE receptors on normodense eosinophils by rosetting? Didn't you report that?

Kay: The impression was that there was more rosetting on hypodense cells than normodense cells.

Capron: I've published experiments comparing different patients and there was no significant difference between hypodense and normodense cells in the proportion of rosettes looking at the different layers, but comparing results from one patient to another patient, we observed huge differences. My hypothesis is that both hypodense and normodense cells can bind IgE through specific binding sites but activation requires something else, probably the epitope which is seen by the monoclonal antibody. We think that our monoclonal antibody binds to a structure which is involved in the activation signal delivered to the cell different from the IgE-binding site. BB10 doesn't bind to the normodense cells.

Kay: I agree with you that there was rosetting with both hypodense and normodense cells and there was a trend for the hypodense to have more rosettes, but they were not significantly different. When we investigated IgA rosettes, we found plenty on neutrophils but not on eosinophils.

Capron: It would be interesting to understand why. Probably because the rosette assay is less sensitive than the fluorescence assay. A very sensitive assay is needed. Secondly, you use normal eosinophils in your IgA rosette assays or did you look also at eosinophils from hypereosinophilic patients?

Kay: Yes, we looked at both. Could I ask you, just on the subject of the binding of immunoglobulins to the surface of the eosinophils. How do you standardize for IgA, IgG, and IgE? How do you know that when you get a negative, you haven't some sort of a prozone effect and you haven't diluted it enough or you shouldn't use more?

Capron: In these kinds of experiments it is important to perform as many measurements as possible. We always compared the FACS analysis with the release of mediators by adding anti-IgE and anti-IgA to cells from all the patients investigated. Only *a posteriori* have we noticed that the cells which have surface IgE or IgA were positive also in the mediator release assay. I have shown you only the two positive patients but we had a lot of patients who were negative. They have normal serum IgE levels and had no surface IgE on eosinophils and these cells were not able to release mediators.

Kay: But, isn't it possible that one range of dilutions may express one mediator production and another range another?

Capron: I agree. We use only two or three doses of each stimulus and the response is very variable depending on the patients, because some may have more surface IgE. We can't use 10 different doses, but our experiments give black or white results, either we have surface immunoglobulins and release or we have no surface immunoglobulins and no release of mediators. We compare the same doses of anti-immunoglobulins, which we know are able to detect surface IgE immunoglobulins.

Makino: Dr Capron, I have one question. You showed anti-IgE and IgG can cause a release of granule specific proteins. Do you think the combination of an anti-IgE and IgG have some enhancing effect?

Capron: It's a good question, because it is the next question we have to answer. What is the relationship between surface IgE and surface IgA versus IgG? We have some preliminary results but it is too soon for discussion. We have indeed observed on some occasions, synergy and on other occasions, decrease effects, when we add two stimuli together.

Spry: Can I first make a comment, then a question. We know that eosinophils have a remarkably long survival in culture under the right conditions, it seems to me that we should not be thinking of eosinophils as similar to neutrophils which come in and do something within half an hour. I think your work is brilliant, since it shows the first steps in the chronic effects of the eosinophils in tissues, which last over days, not over hours. I'll be fascinated to know what kind of secretory events occur when you add the various CSFs, for example, to your cultures and show perhaps prolonged secretion of some newly formed molecules. I think this is the tip of the iceberg and that the eosinophils have a much greater potential. A specific question: do you think there is a close relationship between proteins that you find secreted from eosinophils and the enzymatic properties of the molecules that are secreted? The reason I ask this is that the studies of eosinophil schistosomula binding show lots of peroxidase enzyme present on the surface of the cell. As far as I know, there have been no studies where this enzyme activity has been related in the same EM picture with immuno-localization with a labelled antibody. Is it possible that occasionally these proteins can be secreted in an inactive form? I mean, that might help overcome the problem that you didn't find antigenic EPO.

Capron: Yes, following the results obtained with monoclonal antibodies, I think it's likely that different molecules can be produced under different forms of activation. I think we have to look carefully. For instance, the anti-EPO that we use for the labelling and the electron microscopy is a polyclonal anti-EPO and it would be very interesting to compare results with this antibody with the results using monoclonal anti-EPO antibodies.

Spry: One cannot exclude the secretion of a molecule by the results of a single assay, one must use several assays.

Capron: Yes, absolutely.

Gleich: A very quick comment. Diane McLaren has some rather pretty studies published some time ago showing the deposition of EPO as detected by an enzymatic assay. She associated that with holes in the schistosomula and subsequent invasion of eosinophils through the disrupted tegument. She showed that the peroxidase was at the sites by virtue of its enzymatic activity.

Spry: Yet, the enzyme perhaps could be secreted without being enzymatically active. In those instances where the enzyme is active there is no problem. It's under conditions where you don't see this, as Monique didn't find binding of a particular monoclonal, that the problem arises. It doesn't necessarily mean that activity isn't there and vice versa.

Capron: Yes, I agree.

Kay: Might I add that that was a complement–dependent system which might also explain the difference.

Capron: Yes, it was not the IgE-dependent system at all.

5

Lipid Metabolism by Eosinophils

P. L. B. Bruijnzeel* and J. Verhagen

Department of Pulmonary Disease, State University Utrecht, Utrecht, The Netherlands

5.1 INTRODUCTION

Eosinophils are considered of great importance for the pathogenesis of asthma, since these cells possess the capacity of releasing rather toxic mediators of protein or lipid nature. In this overview the release of various lipid mediators by eosinophils and their significance for the pathogenesis of asthma will be discussed.

In allergic asthmatic individuals allergen provocation may provoke an early phase asthmatic response within 30 min after provocation, as well as a late phase asthmatic response, starting 4–6 h after allergen challenge. The clinically observed reaction pattern of this late phase asthmatic response and the action of certain anti-asthma drugs suggest the involvement of the strongly bronchoconstrictive sulfidopeptide leukotrienes. Together with the finding that eosinophils penetrate into the bronchioli at the beginning of this

---

* Present address: Swiss Institute of Allergy and Asthma Research, Davos, Switzerland.

Eosinophils in Asthma
ISBN 0-12-506452-7

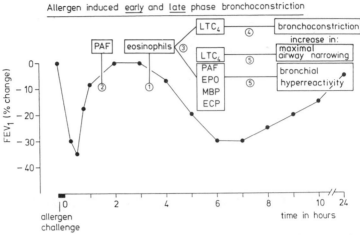

Fig. 1 Schematic representation of our hypothesis concerning the pathogenesis of the allergen-induced late-phase asthmatic reaction (LAR): **1** after an allergen-induced early phase asthmatic reaction sufficient amounts of platelet activating factor (PAF) are generated and released into the circulation to be capable of mobilizing eosinophils in the lung tissue (2); **2** eosinophils do appear in the bronchioli at the beginning of the LAR (1); **3** the infiltrated eosinophils may get activated by as yet unknown substances to release some of its mediators; so far, immune complexes containing IgG (and perhaps IgE) and/or C3b(C3bi), PAF and arachidonic acid seem likely candidates (3); **4** by the release of leukotriene C_4 (LTC_4), the eosinophil may contribute to the broncho-constriction observed during the LAR (4); **5** by the release of eosinophil cationic protein (ECP), major basic protein (MBP), eosinophil peroxidase (EPO) and PAF the bronchial hyperreactivity to methacholine may increase; by the release of LTC_4 the maximal airway narrowing to methacholine may increase. Both these effects are longlasting (5).

reaction, these findings have stimulated us to suggest that eosinophils could actively contribute to this late phase asthmatic reaction by the release of lipid mediators, amongst others sulfidopeptide leukotrienes (1) (Fig. 1). At present, this statement is still hypothetical since there is no clear evidence concerning the *in vivo* release of leukotrienes during this reaction. Moreover, the *in vivo* stimulus for eosinophils to release these mediators remains to be defined.

Here, an overview of the lipid mediators released by eosinophils and their significance for the pathogenesis of asthma will be given.

5.2   ARACHIDONIC ACID METABOLISM IN EOSINOPHILS

After *in vitro* stimulation, human eosinophils are capable of releasing the

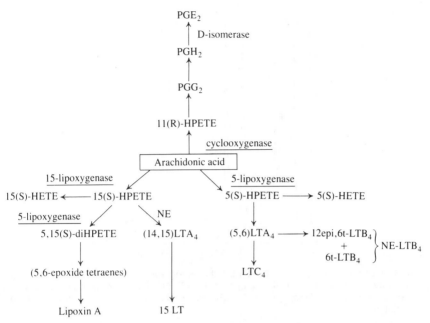

Fig. 2   Schematic representation of the arachidonic acid metabolism of eosinophils (NE; non-enzymatically, NE-LTB$_4$; non-enzymatically formed LTB$_4$).

following arachidonic acid metabolites: prostaglandin E$_2$ (PGE$_2$); leukotriene C$_4$ (LTC$_4$); 15-monohydroxyeicosatetraenoic acid (15-HETE); 15-leukotrienes (15-LT) and lipoxin A (LxA). The release of these arachidonic acid metabolites suggests the presence of cyclooxygenase, 5-lipoxygenase and 15-lipoxygenase activity. The biochemical pathways along which the arachidonic acid metabolites are being formed are outlined in Figure 2.

5.2.1   Cyclooxygenase Pathway in Eosinophils

It has been reported that human eosinophils after *in vitro* challenge with specific allergens and anti-IgE, release an eosinophil derived inhibitor (EDI) of mast cell histamine release (2, 3). This EDI, which pointed out to be a mixture of PGE$_1$ and PGE$_2$, was considered to be a beneficial factor with respect to the allergic reaction process, since it prevented further mast cell degranulation. In our investigations we have incidentally measured the release of PGE$_2$ after *in vitro* challenge of eosinophils with the calcium ionophore A23187 and opsonized zymosan (OZ). The amounts of PGE$_2$ formed ranged from 18–

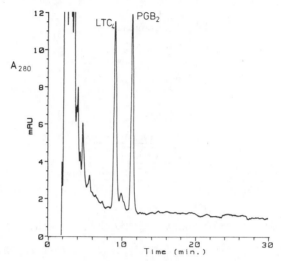

Fig. 3 Illustrative example of a RP-HPLC chromatogram after stimulation of eosinophils (cell purity: 92%) with the calcium ionophore A23187 (10 μ M) in the presence of reduced glutathione (5 mM) for 20 min at 37°C. PGB$_2$ was used as an internal standard. (For technical details see ref. 4.)

77 pg/10^6 cells and were 10^5 times less than the amounts originally reported (2, 3). However, we used different stimuli. Moreover, the specificity of the PGE$_2$ assay has been improved considerably. In comparison with the other lipid mediators to be discussed the quantity of this mediator formed after stimulation seems of little importance.

5.2.2   5-Lipoxygenase Pathway in Eosinophils

5.2.2.1   In vitro *induction of LTC$_4$ formation*

Eosinophils are capable of synthesizing almost exclusively the strongly spasmogenic compound LTC$_4$ when stimulated *in vitro* with the calcium ionophore A23187, OZ, IgG-coated Sepharose particles, PAF or arachidonic acid (4, 5, 6, 7, 8, 9, 10, 11). Figure 3 is an illustrative example of a RP-HPLC profile of the arachidonic acid metabolites formed after stimulation of eosinophils with the calcium ionophore A23187. LTC$_4$ formation induced by all these stimuli was found to be time dependent and completed after 20 min with the calcium ionophore A23187 as a stimulus or after 60 min with the other compounds as stimuli.

Table 1 LTC_4 formation (in $ng/10^6$ cells) by human eosinophils

Stimulus	Concentration	Stimulation time	n	LTC_4
A23187	10 μM	20 min	14	48 ± 7
OZ	2.5 mg/ml	60 min	10	40 ± 8
PAF	10 μM	60 min	31	3.1 ± 0.3
ETE	20 μM	60 min	22	9.2 ± 1.0

Once LTC_4 is formed by the eosinophil it is not further converted into LTD_4 or LTE_4; also added LTC_4 is not metabolized. It has been reported that LTC_4 can be converted into a sulphon or sulphoxide due to the action of eosinophil peroxidase. In our incubations the amounts of these degradation products have been negligible. Since no other sulphidopeptide leukotrienes than LTC_4 are being formed by the eosinophil a LTC_4-radioimmunoassay showing considerable cross-reactivity towards LTD_4 may be used to quantitatively measure the LTC_4 formation. Table 1 summarizes the LTC_4 formation by eosinophils under optimal incubation conditions after stimulation with the calcium ionophore A23187, OZ, PAF or arachidonic acid (ETE).

In the case of stimulation with suboptimal concentrations of the calcium ionophore A23187 and OZ it was observed that LTC_4 release from the cell did not take place immediately. Part of the LTC_4 synthesized remained intracellularly for some time (Fig. 4).

A similar phenomenon has been reported after stimulation with the calcium ionophore A23187 and N-formyl-L-methionyl-L-leucyl-L-phenylalanine (fMLP) (12).

With respect to the pathogenesis of asthma, and in particular the pathogenesis of the allergen-induced late phase asthmatic reaction, the synthesis of LTC_4 by the eosinophil may be of great importance (Fig. 1). Of the above-mentioned stimuli, OZ, PAF and arachidonic acid may be examples of possible in vivo stimuli. So far, our attempts to induce LTC_4 formation via phagocytosis of mast cell granules (from the rat) or via an IgE-mediated process (i.e. after stimulation with Sepharose particles coated with anti-IgE or allergen) have been unsuccessful.

5.2.2.2   Influence of chemotactic factors

Eosinophils are mobilized in the lung tissue via chemotactic factors of protein or lipid nature. As representatives of both groups, fMLP and PAF may be taken. In our incubation system both these compounds were very weak stimuli when used at a concentration up to 1 μM. However, when these

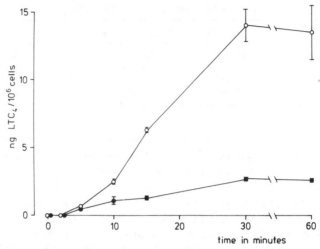

Fig. 4   Intracellular (●) and extracellular (○) LTC_4 after stimulation of eosinophils (cell purity: 87 ± 3%) with opsonized zymosan (OZ, 0.5 mg/ml) in the presence of reduced glutathione (5 mM) at 37°C (mean ± SEM, $n=3$). LTC_4 was extracted from the cell pellets by overnight storage in methanol at 4°C. (For other technical details see ref. 8.)

chemotactic agents were added to some of the stimuli mentioned in Table 1 then a significant increase in LTC_4 formation was induced. This is illustrated in Figure 5.

This synergistic effect may be due to the increase in expression of C3b or Fcγ-receptors (13, 14, 15, 16). On the other hand, these compounds may influence some intracellular processes (e.g. Ca^{2+}-mobilization) which may be of great importance for the final activation of 5-lipoxygenase.

5.2.2.3   Influence of cell-derived mediators

Eosinophils may also be subjected to the influence of cell-derived factors (e.g. monokines, lymphokines), both in the circulation and in the lung tissue. It has been reported that interleukins 1, 3 and 5, granulocyte-macrophage colony-stimulating factor human interferon, a monocyte supernatant and recombinant human tumour necrosis factor do not directly activate the eosinophil but do have the capacity to increase its releasability when it is challenged with another stimulus (40, 18, 19, 20, 21). Since these kind of factors may change the capacity of the eosinophil to release certain mediators considerably we have investigated whether the monocyte supernatant would be capable of increasing the LTC_4 synthesizing capacity after stimulation with

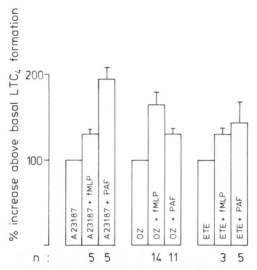

Fig. 5 Amplification of the calcium ionophore A23187 (10 μM), OZ (2.5 mg/ml) and arachidonic acid (ETE, 20 μM) induced LTC$_4$ formation by eosinophils through fMLP (100 nM) and PAF (1 μM). LTC$_4$ synthesis induced by fMLP and PAF was less than 1 ng/10^6 cells. In case of A23187 stimulation the incubation time was 20 min; in case of OZ and ETE stimulation the incubation time was 60 min. The cell purity was generally over 85%. (For absolute values see Table 1; for technical details see refs 8 and 10.)

OZ. This monocyte supernatant is capable of increasing the LTC$_4$ synthesizing capacity of the eosinophil 4–6-fold and is already effective within a pre-incubation of 5 min. This finding corroborates earlier experiments with this monocyte supernatant. It has been reported that this factor is capable of inducing a 2–3-fold increase in the degranulation and the respiratory burst in response to OZ. Furthermore, it causes an almost twofold rise in the expression of C3bi receptors and a transient rise in the intracellular free Ca^{2+} concentration (20). All these effects take place within a pre-incubation time of 5 min. Although this monocyte supernatant has not been further characterized it is thought to have interleukin 1 like properties.

Taken together, these results suggest that, besides chemotactic agents, cell-derived mediators may influence the releasibility of the eosinophil considerably.

5.2.2.4 Influence of cell–cell interaction

Since a great number of chemotactic agents recruit neutrophils and eosino-

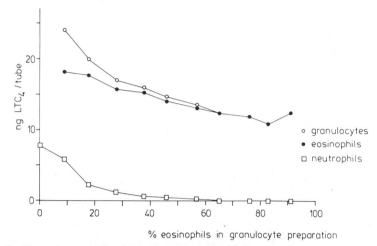

% eosinophils in granulocyte preparation

Fig. 6   Illustrative example of five experiments showing the calcium ionophore A23187 (10 μM) (in the presence of reduced glutathione (5 mM)) induced LTC_4 formation by a granulocyte preparation containing increasing percentages of eosinophils (o) and by a pure neutrophil preparation (containing the same amount of neutrophils as the in the granulocyte preparation) ($\square$). The calculated difference was considered to be the amount of LTC_4 formed by the eosinophils in the granulocyte preparation. The stimulation time in these experiments was 5 min.

phils at the same time, the opportunity exists for cell–cell interaction to occur. This has stimulated us to investigate whether this interaction would influence the LTC_4-synthesizing capacity of the eosinophil. Eosinophils and neutrophils were isolated to almost purity and granulocyte mixtures were prepared which contained increasing percentages of eosinophils. The granulocyte mixture and the amount of pure neutrophils present in this preparation were stimulated and the total amount of LTC_4 formed per tube was measured (Fig. 6). By subtracting the LTC_4 formation of the pure neutrophils from the LTC_4 formation by the granulocyte mixture the LTC_4 formation by the eosinophils could be calculated.

As may be observed in Figure 6, there is an increase in the amount of LTC_4 formed when the granulocyte mixture contains only few eosinophils. It may be speculated that intercellular LTA_4 produced by the neutrophil is responsible for this phenomenon (22). On the other hand, arachidonic acid or some unknown protein factor may be responsible for this effect. Studies are currently being carried out to identify this factor.

This finding may illustrate that besides chemotactic agents and cell-derived mediators also cell–cell interactions can influence the LTC_4 synthesizing capacity of the eosinophils.

5.2.2.5   *LTC₄ formation by eosinophils from peripheral blood of normal and asthmatic individuals*

Supposing that the presence of a blood eosinophilia would indicate activation of this cell type, we have extensively investigated the leukotriene-synthesizing capacity of peripheral blood eosinophils (with identical density) isolated from allergic asthmatic individuals (extrinsic asthmatics), non-allergic asthmatic individuals (intrinsic asthmatics) and age-matched control groups (Fig. 7a, b).

Although one would expect an increased LTC_4 synthesizing capacity when blood eosinophilia is present, no statistically significant differences were observed between the patient groups and the age-matched control groups when the data were corrected for the cell purity of each eosinophil cell preparation investigated. Also when the eosinophils were challenged with OZ, PAF or arachidonic acid, no statistically significant differences were observed between patients and normal controls.

However, some studies (23, 24) have indicated that eosinophils from asthmatic individuals do have a greater capacity to synthesize LTC_4 than the same cells from normal individuals. These findings might be explained by the observation that, in the case of asthmatic individuals, a proportion of the eosinophils in the circulation may possess different characteristics (e.g. lower density, increased metabolic activity) compared with the rest of the eosinophil population (25, 26). Eosinophils with a lower density, so-called hypodense eosinophils, are considered to be metabolically more active than normodense eosinophils. So far, one study has demonstrated that hypodense eosinophils from asthmatic individuals synthesize more LTC_4 than normodense eosinophils (27), whereas another study has demonstrated the complete reverse (28). Our own investigations have never allowed such statements.

5.2.3   15-Lipoxygenase Pathway in Eosinophils

Besides 5-lipoxygenase activity, the eosinophil also exhibits 15-lipoxygenase activity (Fig. 2). (29, 30). In one of our previous studies (5) it has been shown that added arachidonic acid at a concentration over $80\,\mu M$ inhibits the A23187-induced LTC_4 formation (Fig. 8).

RP-HPLC analysis showed that the inhibition of this LTC_4 formation coincided with a striking increase in the synthesis of 15-LTs and 15-HETE. In consecutive experiments, addition of increasing amounts of 15-HETE together with the calcium ionophore A23187 showed a dose dependent inhibi-

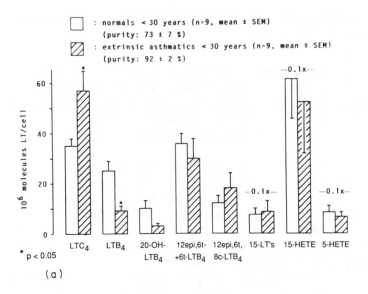

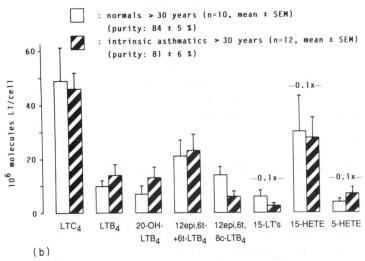

Fig. 7 (a) The calcium ionophore A23187 (10 μM) induced leukotriene formation by human eosinophils isolated from normal individuals and allergic asthmatic individuals (extrinsic asthmatic). (b) The calcium ionophore A23187 (10 μM) induced leukotriene formation by human eosinophils isolated from normal individuals and non-allergic asthmatic individuals (intrinsic asthmatics). (For further technical details see ref. 4.)

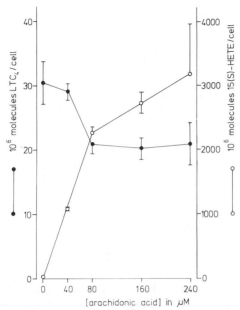

Fig. 8   The effect of added arachidonic acid on the formation of LTC₄ and 15-HETE by isolated human eosinophils ($n=3$, mean $\pm$ SEM). The purity of the eosinophils was 97 $\pm$ 1%. Analysis of LTC₄ was performed by RIA, whereas 15-HETE was analysed by RP-HPLC. (For incubation conditions see ref. 5.)

tion of the LTC$_4$ synthesis (5). Thus, 15-HETE may act as an internal regulator of 5-lipoxygenase activity (5, 31). Interestingly, recent investigations have demonstrated that arachidonic acid itself, without the addition of the calcium ionophore A23187, is capable of inducing LTC$_4$ synthesis, 15-LT and 15-HETE production. At a concentration of arachidonic acid of 50 μM LTC$_4$ formation is slightly inhibited due to the amounts of 15-HETE formed. These findings may be of importance, since it has been reported that 15-HETE is the major arachidonic acid metabolite, especially in human asthmatic lung (32).

With respect to the pathogenesis of asthma the relevance of the formation of 15-LTs and 15-HETE by the eosinophil is not yet clear, although feedback inhibition of 5-lipoxygenase activity seems very important.

5.2.4   Lipoxin A Formation by Human Eosinophils

Lipoxin formation takes place through a combined activity of 15-lipoxyge-

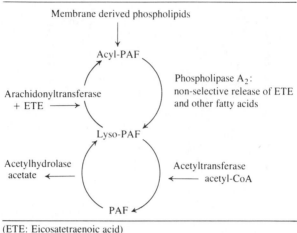

(ETE: Eicosatetraenoic acid)

Fig. 9   PAF biosynthesis by human eosinophils.

nase and 5-lipoxygenase. So far, the following lipoxins have been identified: lipoxin A (LxA); 5(S), 6(R), 15(S)-trihydroxy-7t, 9t, 11c, 13t-eicosatetraenoic acid and lipoxin B (LxB); 5(S), 14(R), 15(S)-trihydroxy-6t, 8c, 10t, 12t-eicosatetraenoic acid (33, 34, 35).

Quite recently, LxA formation by the human eosinophil has been reported when challenged with the calcium ionophore A23187 (2.5 μM) in the presence of arachidonic acid at a concentration of 80 μM (36). The amount of LxA formed was 20–50 times less than the amount of LTC$_4$ formed, since stimulation of eosinophils by the calcium ionophore A23187, together with arachidonic acid, may induce the formation of considerable amounts of 15-HETE (Fig. 8) it may be possible that the activated eosinophils utilize 15-HETE to generate LxA.

At present it is not yet clear how LxA would be involved in the pathogenesis of asthma. Nevertheless, it has been reported that LxA, among others, may stimulate neutrophils to degranulate (33), may inhibit human natural killer cell function (37) and has contractile activity (38).

5.3   PLATELET ACTIVATING FACTOR FORMATION BY HUMAN EOSINOPHILS

The biosynthesis of platelet activating factor (PAF) is outlined in Figure 9. It

Table 2   Effects of lipid mediators released by eosinophils

Mediator	Effect
PGE_2	Inhibition of mast cell degranulation
LTC_4	Contraction of smooth muscle; oedema and mucus production
15-HETE	Chemotaxis of granulocytes; inhibition of 5-lipoxygenase activity in eosinophils
lipoxin A	Degranulation of granulocytes; inhibition of natural killer cell cytotoxicity
PAF	Chemotaxis of granulocytes; induction of bronchial hyperreactivity

has been shown that eosinophils do have the capacity to synthesize this very potent lipid mediator (39). However, the amounts synthesized are at least a 1000-fold less than the amounts of LTC_4 synthesized under the same incubation conditions. On the contrary, it has been demonstrated that eosinophils obtained from the bronchoalveolar lavage fluid of asthmatic individuals have the capacity, upon challenge with allergen or anti-IgE, to release amounts of PAF similar to the ones observed for LTC_4 (M. Capron, pers. comm.). Whether these eosinophils have been altered by environmental factors, present in the lung tissue, remains to be elucidated. At any rate, more evidence is needed to prove that PAF release from intact eosinophils occurs and seriously contributes to the pathogenesis of asthma.

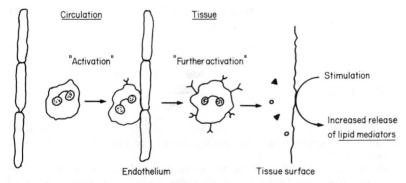

Fig. 10   Eosinophils may get primed or activated in the circulation by certain chemotactic factors, cell-derived mediators and cell–cell interactions. Further activation may take place when the eosinophils migrate into the tissue. Moreover, certain surface receptors may be expressed facilitating final stimulation. These eosinophils are easily triggered to release their mediators.

5.4   CONCLUDING REMARKS

This paper has given an overview of the lipid mediators released by eosinophils. Table 2 summarizes some of the effects of those mediators which may have significance for the pathogenesis of asthma. According to the literature, LTC_4 and 15-HETE are the most abundant arachidonic acid metabolites *in vitro*. However, these data may not reflect the *in vivo* situation. Data have therefore been presented to underline that chemotactic agents, cell-derived mediators and cell–cell interactions may change the capacity of the eosinophil to release certain lipid mediators. Moreover, when eosinophils migrate from the circulation into the tissue, the expression of certain surface receptors may be induced or increased. Thus, the releasibility of the eosinophil reaching the tissue surface may be have changed completely compared with the eosinophil in the circulation. A scheme of the possible events taking place when eosinophils migrate into the tissue is shown in Figure 10.

Based on this scheme future investigations should focus on how environmental factors, present in the circulation and the lung tissue change the expression of surface receptors on the eosinophil and the capacity of the eosinophil to release certain mediators, in particular lipid mediators.

Acknowledgements

The authors wish to thank Mr P. T. M. Kok, Mrs M. L. Hamelink and Mrs G. M. Kijne for skilled technical assistance. Part of these investigations were financially supported by the Dutch Asthma Foundation grants 82.18 and 86.36.

REFERENCES

1. Bruijnzeel, P. L. B., Verhagen, J. (1989). The possible role of particular leukotrienes in the allergen-induced late phase asthmatic reaction. *Clin. Exp. Allergy* **19**, Suppl. 1, 25–32.
2. Hubscher, T. (1975). Role of the eosinophil in the allergic reactions. I. EDI—An eosinophil-derived inhibitor of histamine release. *J. Immunol.* **144**, 1379–1388.
3. Hubscher, T. (1975). Role of the eosinophil in the allergic reactions. II. Release of prostaglandins from human eosinophil leukocytes. *J. Immunol.* **114**, 1389–1393.

4. Verhagen, J., Bruijnzeel, P. L. B., Koedam, J. A., Wassink, G. A., de Boer, M., Terpstra, G. K., Kreukniet, J., Veldink, G. A., Vliegenthart, J. F. G. (1984). Specific leukotriene formation by purified human eosinophils and neutrophils. *FEBS Lett.* **168**, 23–28.

5. Bruijnzeel, P. L. B., Kok, P. T. M., Viëtor, R. J., Verhagen, J. (1984). On the optimal conditions of LTC_4 formation by human eosinophils *in vitro*. *Prostagl. leukotr. Med.* **20**, 11–22.

6. Weller, P. F., Lee, C. W., Foster, D. W., Corey, E. J., Austen, K. F., Lewis, R. A. (1983). Generation and metabolism of 5-lipoxygenase pathway leukotrienes by human eosinophils: predominant production of leukotriene C_4. *Proc. Natl. Acad. Sci. USA* **80**, 7626–7630.

7. Shaw, R. J., Cromwell, O., Kay, A. B. (1984). Preferential generation of leukotriene C_4 by human eosinophils. *Clin. Exp. Immunol.* **56**, 716–722.

8. Bruijnzeel, P. L. B., Kok, P. T. M., Hamelink, M. L., Kijne, G. M., Verhagen, J. (1985). Exclusive leukotriene C_4 synthesis by purified human eosinophils induced by opsonized zymosan. *FEBS Lett.* **189**, 350–354.

9. Shaw, R. J., Walsh, G. M., Cromwell, O., Moqbel, R., Spry, C. J. F., Kay, A. B. (1985). Activated human eosinophils generate SRS-A leukotrienes following IgG-dependent stimulation. *Nature* **316**, 150–152.

10. Bruijnzeel, P. L. B., Kok, P. T. M., Hamelink, M. L., Kijne, G. M., Verhagen, J. (1986). Platelet activating factor induces leukotriene C_4 synthesis by purified human eosinophils. *Prostaglandins* **34**, 205–214.

11. Kok, P. T. M., Hamelink, M. L., Kÿne, G. M., Verhagen, J., Koenderman, L., Bruijnzeel, P. L. B. (1988). Arachidonic acid can induce leukotriene C_4 formation by purified human eosinophils in the absence of other stimuli. *Biochem. Biophys. Res. Comm.* **153**, 676–682.

12. Owen, W. F., Soberman, R. J., Yochimoto, T., Sheffer, A. L., Lewis, R. A., Austen, F. K. (1987). Synthesis and release of leukotriene C_4 by human eosinophils. *J. Immunol.* **138**, 532–538.

13. Anwar, A. R. E., Kay, A. B. (1977). The ECF-A tetrapeptides and histamine selectively enhance human eosinophil complement receptors. *Nature* **269**, 522–524.

14. Capron, M. A., Capron, A., Goetzl, E. J., Austen, K. F. (1981). Eosinophil Fc receptor: Enhancement by the tetrapeptides of the eosinophil chemotactic factor of anaphylaxis (ECF-A). *Nature* **289**, 71–73.

15. Kay, A. B., Walsh, G. M. (1984). Chemotactic factor-induced enhancement of the binding of human immunoglobulin classes and subclasses to neutrophils and eosinophils. *Clin. Exp. Immunol.* **57**, 729–734.

16. Nagy, L., Lee, T. H., Goetzl, E. J., Pickett, W. C., Kay, A. B. (1982). Complement receptor enhancement and chemotaxis of human neutrophils and eosinophils by leukotrienes and other lipoxygenase products. *Clin. Exp. Immunol.* **47**, 541–547.

17. Pincus, S. H., Whitcomb, E. A., Dinarello, C. A. (1986). Interaction of IL1 and TPA in modulation of eosinophil function. *J. Immunol.* **137**, 3509–3514.

18. Lopez, A. F., Sanderson, C. J., Gamble, J. R., Campbell, H. D., Young, I. G., Vadas, M. E. (1988). Recombinant human interleukin 5 is a selective activator of human eosinophil function. *J. Exp. Med.* **167**, 219–224.

19. Saito, H., Hayakawa, T., Yui, Y., Shida, T. (1987). Effect of human interferon on different functions of human neutrophils and eosinophils. *Int. Archs. Allergy appl. Immun.* **82**, 133–140.

20. Yazdanbakhsh, M. (1987). "Immunobiology of eosinophils", pp. 121–141. Thesis, Amsterdam.
21. Roubin, R., Elsas, P. P., Fiers, W., Dessein, A. J. (1987). Recombinant human tumour necrosis factor (rTNF)[2] enhances leukotriene biosynthesis in neutrophils and eosinophils stimulated with the Ca^{2+} ionophore A23187. *Clin. Exp. Immunol.* **70**, 484–490.
22. Feinmark, S. J., Cannon, P. J. (1986). Endothelial cell leukotriene C_4 synthesis results from intercellular transfer of leukotriene A_4 synthesized by polymorphonuclear leukocytes. *J. Biol. Chem.* **261**, 16466–16472.
23. Mita, H., Yui, Y., Taniguchi, N., Yasueda, H., Shida, T. (1985). Increased activity of 5-lipoxygenase in polymorphonuclear leukocytes from asthmatic patients. *Life Sci.* **37**, 907–914.
24. Mita, H., Yui, Y., Yasueda, H., Kajita, T., Saito, H., Shida, T. (1986). Allergen-induced histamine release and immunoreactive leukotriene C_4 generation from leukocytes in mite sensitive asthmatic patients. *Prostaglandins* **31**, 869–886.
25. Prin, L., Capron, M., Tonnel, A. B., Bletry, O., Capron, A. (1983). Heterogeneity of human peripheral blood eosinophils. Variability in cell density and cytotoxic ability in relation to the level and the origin of hypereosinophilia. *Int. Archs. Allergy appl. Immun.* **72**, 336–346.
26. Winqvist, I., Olofsson, T., Olsson, I., Persson, A. M., Hallberg, T. (1982). Altered density, metabolism and surface receptors of eosinophils in eosinophilia. *Immunology* **47**, 531–539.
27. Kajita, T., Yui, Y., Mita, H., Taniguchi, N., Saito, H., Mishima, T., Shida, T. (1985). Release of leukotriene C_4 from human eosinophils and its relation to the cell density. *Int. Archs. Allergy appl. Immun.* **78**, 406–410.
28. Kauffman, H. F., van der Belt, B., de Monchy, J. G. R., Boelens, H., Koëter, G. H., de Vries, K. (1987). Leukotriene C_4 production by normal-density and low-density eosinophils of atopic individuals and other patients with eosinophilia. *J. Allergy Clin. Immunol.* **79**, 611–619.
29. Turk, J., Maas, R. L., Brash, A. R., Roberts, J., Oates, J. A. (1982). Arachidonic acid 15-lipoxygenase products from human eosinophils. *J. Biol. Chem.* **257**, 7068–7076.
30. Henderson, W. R., Harley, J. B., Fauci, A. S. (1984). Arachidonic acid metabolism in normal and hypereosinophilic syndrome human eosinophils: generation of leukotrienes B_4, C_4, D_4 and 15-lipoxygenase products. *Immunology* **51**, 679–686.
31. Van der Hoek, J. Y., Bryant, R. W., Bailey, J. M. (1980). Inhibition of leukotriene biosynthesis by the leukocyte product 15-hydroxy-5, 8, 11, 13-eicosatetraenoic acid. *J. Biol. Chem.* **225**, 10064–10065.
32. Hamberg, M., Hedqvist, P., Radegran, K. (1980). Identification of 15-hydroxy-5, 8, 11, 13-eicosatetraenoic acid (15-HETE) as a major metabolite of arachidonic acid in human lung. *Acta Physiol. Scand.* **110**, 219–221.
33. Serhan, C. N., Hamberg, M., Samuelsson, B. (1984). Lipoxins: Novel series of biologically active compounds formed from arachidonic acid in human leukocytes. *Proc. Natl. Acad. Sci. USA* **81**, 5335–5339.
34. Serhan, C. N., Nicolaou, K. C., Webber, S. E., Veale, C. A., Dahlén, S-E., Puustinen, T. J., Samuelsson, B. (1986). Lipoxin A: Stereochemistry and biosynthesis. *J. Biol. Chem.* **26**, 16340–16345.
35. Serhan, C. N., Hamberg, M., Samuelsson, B., Morris, J., Whiska, D. G. (1986). On

the stereochemistry and biosynthesis of lipoxin B. *Proc. Natl. Acad. Sci. USA* **83**, 1983–1987.

36. Serhan, C. N., Hirsch, U., Palmblad, J., Samuelsson, B. (1987). Formation of lipoxin A by granulocytes from eosinophilic donors. *FEBS Lett.* **217**, 242–246.
37. Ramstedt, U., Serhan, C. N., Nicolaou, K. C., Webber, S. E., Wigzell, H., Samuelsson, B. (1987). Lipoxin A-induced inhibition of human natural killer cell cytotoxicity: studies on stereospecificity of inhibition and mode of action. *J. Immunol.* **138**, 266–270.
38. Rokach, J., Fitzsimmons, B. J., Adams, J., Evans, J. F., Leblanc, Y. (1986). The lipoxins: determination of their biosynthesis. *Pharmacol. Res. Comm.* **18**, 11–23.
39. Lee, T. C., Lenihan, D. J., Malone, B., Roddy, L. L., Wasserman, S. I. (1984). Increased biosynthesis of platelet-activating factor in activated human eosinophils. *J. Biol. Chem.* **259**, 5526–5530.
40. Silberstein, D. S., David, J. R. (1987). The regulation of human eosinophil function by cytokines. *Immunol. Today* **12**, 380–385.

After preparation of this manuscript a publication appeared (Parsons and Roberts, *J. Immunol.* (1988) **141**, 2413–2419) which described that the main cyclooxygenase product formed by peripheral blood eosinophils, upon challenge with the calcium ionophore A23187, was thromboxane B_2 (2247 pg/10^6 eosinophils), whereas only small amounts of PGE_2 (483 pg/10^6 eosinophils), $PGF_{2\alpha}$ (265 pg/10^6 eosinophils) and PGD_2 (50 pg/10^6 eosinophils) were synthesized. Compared with the lipoxygenase products formed these amounts are still relatively small.

DISCUSSION

Makino (Chairman): What was your source of eosinophils?

Bruijnzeel: We use blood from normal individuals in most studies. We obtain buffy-coats from 500 ml of blood of those individuals (via the blood transformation laboratory) from which we can isolate eosinophils at purity over 85%. If we use asthmatic individuals, we need only 100 ml of blood.

Vargaftig: You've shown some interesting data on the modulation of the release of leukotriene C_4 and 15-HETE with arachidonic acid under the conditions which suggested that arachidonic acid might be involved. Have you substantiated your results by doing experiments in the presence of indomethacin or aspirin or replacing arachidonic acid with PGE_2? One of the problems with arachidonic acid, as you know, is that it goes everywhere and that it is transformed into products that do everything.

Bruijnzeel: We have not performed these experiments. I agree with you that we should perform them.

Vargaftig: I have another question. It's about the relatively negative data on PAF in one of your slides. I noticed that you found some PAF in the pellet. A lot of work, particularly from Pinckard's group, has shown that most PAF remains on the cell, and is not secreted. Did you do experiments in which you measured lyso-PAF by detecting PAF following reacetylation? It is possible that an acetylhydrolase has been active, so you would never find PAF, only lyso-PAF.

Bruijnzeel: We have not carried out re-acetylation experiments.

Vargaftig: I think that it's very important to substantiate any claim for negative data.

Makino: This is a very important point. Many cells produce PAF but frequently we couldn't find PAF in our supernatants.

Wasserman: It's interesting that you find that the chemotactic tripeptide synergizes with other stimuli for leukotriene production, because a number of groups are advocating pre-treating blood cells with the tripeptide to enable separation of eosinophils from neutrophils. Whilst that separation may work, this result suggests that it may yield an altered eosinophil preparation.

Bruijnzeel: I'm glad you have raised that point. Most of my isolations, as perhaps you know, use fMLP. In the original report of Roberts and Gallin, 10^{-6} molar fMLP was used for isolating the eosinophils in a one-step procedure, using discontinuous gradient centrifugation on Percoll. It has been clearly shown by Maria Yazdanbakhsh that this concentration causes activation of eosinophils. In the same paper, it was also shown that 10^{-8} molar fMLP primed eosinophils for a subsequent stimulation. But if you use a calcium-free medium with this low fMLP concentration, then eosinophils are not activated in a measurable way. Of course, you have to use normal eosinophils.

Wasserman: It is possible that you see no synergy between fMLP and the calcium ionophore, because they are both inducing increased calcium concentrations within the cell. Another point, relating to PAF production and the identification of PAF within the pellet and not in the supernatant—most of the studies on neutrophils, and I know the controversy about the number of cells in the experiments, were done by Peter Henson's group and they are very adamant about the fact that PAF is not released from neutrophils. Professor Benveniste feels that if the number of neutrophils are decreased dramatically, one then begins to appreciate PAF in the supernatants. Your data look very much like our data on PAF production by eosinophils. The most potent stimulus for generation of PAF was the calcium ionophore, but the most potent stimuli for release of PAF were the soluble chemotactic factors.

Kay: Peter, I enjoyed your talk. We are doing similar experiments and have measured PAF generation by hypodense, normal- and light-density eosinophils and also neutrophils, cells which were kindly supplied to us by Christopher Spry. The experiments that Stephen Wasserman referred to from his own group, I think detected fmole amounts of PAF and in our experiments we are getting nanogram amounts per million cells. That is nothing like the hundreds of nanograms that Monique Capron and Jacques Benveniste seem to be getting from an IgE stimulus, but I think the amounts are quite substantial. fmet-leu-phe does increase the amount of PAF in the supernatant, but the dose response is not perfect. Normal eosinophils seem to be much better at producing PAF than hypodense cells or neutrophils. I think it's important to distinguish between normal and hypodense eosinophils, particularly in the monocyte supernatant experiments. We've found, using Anthony Butterworth's factor, the light-density cells were quite unresponsive, only the normal-density cells produced PAF. Normal-density cells generate about five times more PAF and that's following stimulation with the ionophore as well as IgG-coated beads. The normal density cells seem to have increased amounts of extracellular PAF following pretreatment. PAF seems to be retained by the light-density cells.

Makino: You have shown co-culture with the monocyte supernatant or co-culture with neutrophils enhance the LTC_4 production by eosinophils. So do you have any idea what is the factor which enhances the LTC_4 production?

Bruijnzeel: This is in some way speculative but the work of Maria Yazdanbakhsh has shown that the monocyte supernatant has the capacity to mobilize cytosolic calcium intracellularly. The lipoxygenase activity needs calcium, so this may explain the increased release of LTC_4 after challenge with opsonized zymosan. I think the other point on the interaction between neutrophils and eosinophils is a very intriguing one, because we don't know which factor passes from neutrophils to the eosinophils. It was suggested that LTA_4 may move through the membrane and serve as kind of substrate. So that may be one explanation. We are doing experiments to find out which factor is indeed released.

Vadas: I have just a couple of questions to ask. Firstly, about a monocyte factor. I remember a paper by Silberstein and David, Journal of Immunology about a year ago; didn't they show that GM-CSF enhances LTC_4 production?

Bruijnzeel: Yes, that's right.

Vadas: I think that GM-CSF ought to be acknowledged as a cloned product that works, and, therefore, hypotheses about other factors have to be based on some other evidence. The second point I'd like to make relates to neutrophil contamination. I think that probably it is an oversimplification, because your methods of purification leave platelets behind. We've spent an enormous amount of time comparing about five different ways of purification to remove platelets and the only one that gives you any chance of getting rid of them is elutriation. Unless you use elutriation, you have ten platelets per granulocyte at the minimum. Without specifically looking at the effects of removing the platelets, it is just an hypothesis that it is the neutrophils which are involved in the cellular interaction. It is necessary to control for the platelets.

Bruijnzeel: Yes, I agree with that. We have not controlled the presence of platelets. But, people working in the microbiology department use the same isolation procedure for granulocytes and they have checked preparations with electron microscopy. They report an average of three platelets per granulocyte.

Vargaftig: I would like to make a comment on the interaction between f Met-Leu-Phe and the eosinophil. We have a paper in press demonstrating that even though the human eosinophil, at least in our hands, was relatively poorly reactive to f Met-Leu-Phe *in vitro*, the *in vivo* situation is completely different.

If you inject f Met-Leu-Phe into the human arm of an allergic patient, you obtain more or less the same result as that achieved with PAF. There is a major invasion of eosinophils, one-third of which are degranulated. So, either it's a direct effect, which you lose when you do *in vitro* experiments, or there is something coming in between.

Bruijnzeel: Perhaps I may comment on that. In relation to the isolation procedure, we have challenged eosinophils with f Met-Leu-Phe. If you have very pure eosinophils and you determine the dose response with f Met-Leu-Phe, 10^{-6} M causes leukotriene C_4 formation whilst at 10^{-8} M no synthesis of LTC_4 or eosinophil activation is observed. However, when you add neutrophils, which don't release LTC_4, to the eosinophils, then there is an enhancement by a factor of 2 or 3 with respect to the LTC_4 formation, suggesting perhaps an interaction between eosinophils and neutrophils. The involvement of platelets and PAF must not be neglected and needs investigation.

Kay: First of all, I think in all these experiments the interesting thing is that the eosinophils are producing so much LTC_4, whereas the neutrophils and the monocytes produce much less. If it's a platelet problem, then the platelets must preferentially go with the eosinophils and I don't think there is any evidence for that, although it's an important point. The other comment relates to the work of Bill Henderson. He has shown very elegantly that neutrophils do have the capacity for producing LTC_4 and that they rapidly metabolize it through their MPO system, because in MPO deficient patients neutrophils can produce appreciable amounts of LTC_4. Neutrophils also produce LTC_4 if the activity of MPO is blocked. I think it's still an open question as to what is the reason you get LTB_4 with neutrophils and LTC_4 with eosinophils. Is it due to the lack of an enzyme or pathway or, as Bill Henderson has proposed, due to increased metabolism?

Bruijnzeel: I have no answer to that question. Investigation of the calcium ionophore-induced leukotriene C_4 synthesis by different combinations of neutrophils and eosinophils showed that almost pure neutrophils with 3% eosinophils, when challenged for five minutes, synthesize leukotriene C_4. So, there must be some factor which triggers in neutrophils the capacity to synthesize leukotriene C_4. Vice versa, under certain circumstances when you add arachidonic acid, eosinophils get the capacity to synthesize LTB_4. One can speculate that if you augment the LTA_4 in the cells, then you probably trigger further pathways.

Dahl: The hypothesis that the eosinophil goes from the bloodstream to the tissues and stays there may explain the differences observed between blood eosinophils and lavage eosinophils for example. But I thought there were data which showed that eosinophils would move freely back and forward from the blood stream to the tissues. Such freedom of movement would require a different theory.

Bruijnzeel: Yes, I agree with that.

Capron: I have a question about PAF. I'm pleased, Dr Kay, that your results show that normodense cells produce PAF after IgG stimulation, whereas my results show that hypodense cells produce PAF after IgE stimulation, which fits well with the cytotoxic function of IgG versus IgE. A first question: did you look at the differences in subclasses of IgG when you stimulated your normodense eosinophils? And the second question: did you look at the production of lyso-PAF? Looking at the production of PAF in the IgE stimulation of hypodense cells, we were surprised to observe that stimulation of hypodense cells by IgG produced lyso-PAF and not PAF.

Kay: No, we haven't looked at the IgG subclasses but I doubt that they would be different, because of the nature of the binding to eosinophils and neutrophils of the Fc receptors. We haven't measured lyso-PAF. We also observed that light density eosinophils can produce LTC_4 through an IgE-dependent mechanism in a schistosomulum system.

Spry: This is a question for clarification. In the literature, LTC_4 production always seems to require added arachidonic acid but you have shown quite good LTC_4 release without any added arachidonic acid. Can you clarify that and also explain how in aspirin-sensitive patients the eosinophils could be releasing LTC_4. Is there an important message in that clinical story?

Bruijnzeel: In our stimulation system we add reduced glutathione as well as calcium and we don't need to add arachidonic acid. The original reports from the Swedes used arachidonic acid but Professor Kay as well as Peter Weller have shown that you don't need arachidonic acid to have leukotriene C_4 production, so probably the intracellular stored pool is high enough. A recent publication from Germany showed that fMLP and PAF stimulation release intracellular arachidonic acid but only a part is used for LTC_4 production, whereas calcium ionophore stimulation uses all the arachidonic acid which is released. This may explain the differences in amounts of LTC_4 produced although the amounts of arachidonic acid released intracellularly are almost the same.

Spry: And the other was the aspirin story.

Bruijnzeel: I only showed you the results with the extrinsic allergic asthmatic patients, but we have compared these data with those of intrinsic asthmatic patients, who have no positive skin tests or IgE. Most of these patients have eosinophilia but the eosinophils have the same density as the normal eosinophils and synthesize the same amounts of LTC_4. I think Professor Kay has similar data.

Kay: The validity of feeding exogenous arachidonic acid calls into question many experiments, including not only lipid mediated production of leukotrienes by eosinophils but also epithelial cells.

6

Role of Eosinophil Chemotactic Factors on Eosinophil Activation and Leukotriene C$_4$ Production

N. Tamura, D. K. Agrawal and R. G. Townley

Allergic Disease Center,
Creighton University School of Medicine,
Omaha, Nebraska 68178, USA

6.1 INTRODUCTION

Several possible mechanisms have been proposed to explain airway hyper-reactivity (1). However, the precise mechanism is still unclear. Recently, the possibility has been increasingly recognized that the accumulation of inflammatory cells in the airway and the chemical mediators released from these cells are important factors for the development of inflammatory pulmonary diseases (2). Many of the chemical mediators have been identified and thought to be at least a part of the mechanisms of pulmonary inflammation (3). Among these chemical mediators, leukotriene (LTC$_4$, LTD$_4$ and LTE$_4$)

Eosinophils in Asthma
ISBN 0-12-506452-7

the constituents of the slow-reacting substance of anaphylaxis, induce potent and prolonged airway constriction which differs from that induced by histamine (4–6).

Platelet activating factor (PAF), a phospholipid mediator, is released from a variety of inflammatory cells including basophils, platelets, neutrophils, macrophages and eosinophils (7–11). PAF in turn possesses significant effects on these cells both *in vitro* and *in vivo* (12). Local administration of PAF induces cell infiltration including neutrophils (13) and eosinophils (14), and these observations imply that PAF works as a chemotactic factor. On the other hand, PAF causes the extravasation of blood components (15), and this could be the reason for the cellular accumulation. In fact, it has been reported that PAF is a potent neutrophil chemotactic factor *in vitro* (16). However, there is no convincing study as yet on the effect of PAF on purified eosinophils.

The accumulation of eosinophils in the bronchial tissue is one of the characteristics seen in bronchial asthma patients, and the evidence for the contribution of eosinophils to the pathogenesis of bronchial asthma is increasing (17, 18). The contribution of eosinophils may be mainly attributed to two different mechanisms: the injurious effect on the bronchial tree by eosinophil granule proteins; and the bronchoconstriction induced by LTC_4 produced from eosinophils.

Eosinophils are known to produce LTC_4 predominantly and preferentially when stimulated by calcium ionophore (19–21) and by immune complexes (22). Wang *et al.* (23) reported increased LTC_4 production from leukocytes in bronchial asthma patients. Kauffman *et al.* (24) reported the difference in LTC_4 production between hypodense and normodense eosinophils, and Fukuda *et al.* (25) reported increased proportion of hypodense eosinophils in bronchial asthma patients.

De Monchy *et al.* (26) recently, reported bronchoalveolar eosinophilia and elevated eosinophil cationic protein in the bronchoalveolar fluid during late asthmatic response. Metzger *et al.* (27) reported the generation of eosinophil chemotactic activity during early and late asthmatic responses after antigen challenge. Many of the factors which attract eosinophils to the inflammatory site have been reported (28). It has been reported very recently that PAF is a potent chemotactic factor for eosinophils in patients with hypereosinophilia (29) and in normal subjects (30). After the induction of chemotaxis, eosinophil chemotactic factor of anaphylaxis (ECF-A) (31) and PAF (30) induce the deactivation of eosinophils for further chemotaxis. However, very little is known about the role and the mechanism of eosinophil chemotactic factors on eosinophil functions after the induction of chemotaxis.

In this study, therefore, we evaluated the direct chemotactic effect and the modifying effects of naturally occurring eosinophil chemotactic factors (PAF, ECF-A and LTB_4) on the LTC_4 production from eosinophils, and hypothesized the possible mechanisms of these eosinophil chemotactic factors in the inflammatory processes.

6.2 METHODS

6.2.1 Subjects

Twenty-two subjects (10 healthy subjects, 8 mild allergic bronchial asthma patients, 3 allergic rhinitis patients and 1 atopic dermatitis patient) participated in this study. The age of the subjects ranged from 20 to 40 years (average 29.3 yrs), and the distribution of the sex was 18 males and 4 females. The mean white blood cell count was $5797/mm^3$, and the percentage of eosinophil was $3.9 \pm 0.5\%$ (the mean $\pm$ SEM) (range 1.4–9.4%). The patients were without any symptoms at the time blood was drawn. Blood was obtained between 8 and 11 A.M. None of the subjects was taking corticosteroids or any other medications during the month prior to this study except inhaled bronchodilators. The study was approved by the Human Experimental Committee of Creighton University School of Medicine.

6.2.2 Reagents, materials and buffers

Synthetic PAF (C16) and lyso-PAF (C16) were purchased from Bachem Fine Chemicals (Torrance, CA), dissolved in ethyl alcohol as a stock solution, and stored at $-70°C$ until use. Synthetic LTB_4 was a gift from Dr J. Rokach (Merck Frosst Canada Inc., Pointe Claire, Quebec, Canada), dissolved in methyl alcohol and stored at $-70°C$. L-alanylglycyl-l-seryl-l-glutamic acid (ECF-A), phorbol 12-myristate 13-acetate (PMA), cytochalasin B, calcium ionophore A23187, human serum albumin factor V, colloidal polyvinylpyrrolidone coated silica gel (Percoll), ficoll-sodium diatrizoate (Histopaque), n-2-hydroxyethylpiperazine-n'-2-ethanesulfonic acid (HEPES), dextran (M.W. 506 000) and l-phosphatidyl-l-serine were purchased from Sigma Chemical Co. (St. Louis, MO). Ethylenediaminetetraacetate (EDTA), sodium borate, methylene blue, Wright's stain solution, a hydrometer and 12 × 75 mm borosilicated glass tubes were purchased from Fisher Scientific Co. (Fair Lawn, NJ). A radioimmunoassay kit specific for LTC_4 was purchased from Amersham Corp. (Arlington Heights, IL). Hanks' balanced salt solution (HBSS) without Ca^{2+}, Mg^{2+} and $NaHCO_3$, and 0.4% trypan blue solution were obtained from GIBCO (Grand Island, NY). 15 ml polystyrene conical centrifugation tubes were purchased from Corning Glass Ware (Corning, NY).

Buffers used in this study were as follows; phosphate buffered saline (NaCl 137.0 mM, KCl 2.7 mM, Na_2HPO_4 8.0 mM and KH_2PO_4 1.5 mM, pH 7.4), modified HBSS (supplemented with $CaCl_2$ 1.8 mM, $MgCl_2.6H_2O$ 1.0 mM, $NaHCO_3$ 4.2 mM and HEPES 9.7 mM, pH 7.4), and the incubation buffer (NaCl 120.0 mM, KCl 5.4 mM, $CaCl_2$ 1.8 mM, $MgCl_2.6H_2O$ 1.0 mM, KH_2PO_4 0.4 mM, $NaHCO_3$ 4.2 mM, l-serine 5.0 mM, sodium borate 10.0 mM, HEPES 9.7 mM, glucose 5.0 mM and 0.25% human serum albumin, pH 7.4). Each reagent used in the study was finally dissolved in the incubation buffer.

6.2.3   Separation of Eosinophils

A purified eosinophil fraction was obtained according to the method previously described (30) with modifications. Forty millilitres of venous blood was drawn into a syringe containing anticoagulant (1 ml of 2% sodium-EDTA/10 ml of whole blood). Anti-coagulated blood was then sedimented with 6% dextran in normal saline (4 vol of blood/1 vol of dextran solution) for 60 min at room temperature. The plasma-leukocyte fraction was collected, diluted with phosphate buffered saline and washed twice by centrifugation (400 × g for 10 min at 4°C). Leukocytes were suspended in 10 ml of modified HBSS.

Eosinophils were separated by discontinuous density gradient centrifugation. The mixtures of Percoll (density = 1.130) and Histopaque (density = 1.077) were prepared to obtain final densities of 1.085 and 1.081. Each density was determined using a hydrometer at 20°C. The osmolarity of the mixtures ranged from 270 to 290 mosm/kg H_2O as determined by freezing-point depression. Four-and-a-half millilitres of the heavier mixture (d = 1.085) was placed into the bottom of a 15 ml conical centrifugation tube, and 1.5 ml of the lighter mixture (d = 1.081) and 2 ml of Histopaque were then carefully overlayered. Then 5 ml of the leukocyte suspension was applied on the density gradient. After centrifugation (700 × g for 35 min at room temperature), three distinct bands and a pellet were obtained. All bands (comprising neutrophils, mononuclear cells and a small percentage of eosinophils) and the density gradient mixtures were removed carefully by aspiration. The pellet (d = 1.085) consisted of eosinophils (87.1 ± 2.4%), neutrophils (12.8 ± 2.1%) and a small number of red blood cells. We considered the eosinophils obtained as normodense eosinophils (25). After obtaining the eosinophil fraction, red blood cells were removed by hypotonic lysis, and washed twice by centrifugation ($400 \times g$ for 10 min at $4°C$) in modified HBSS. Finally, eosinophils were suspended in the incubation buffer at a concentration from 1.0 to 3.0×10^6 eosinophils/ml.

Leukocyte count and the purity of eosinophils were confirmed by Randolph stain (32) with methylene blue and/or Wright's stain. The cell viability was evaluated by trypan blue dye exclusion, and was always greater than 96%.

6.2.4 Chemotactic Experiment

Chemotactic experiments were performed using modified Boyden chambers and 3 μm pore size polycarbonate filters.

A specified concentration of either PAF, ECF-A or LTB₄ in 200 μl HBSS was placed in the lower compartment of the chamber and 2×10^5 eosinophils were applied into the upper compartment. As a control, the lower compartment contained only HBSS. Both the upper and lower compartments contained the same concentration of the stimulus as for chemokinetic experiments. Chemotactic, chemokinetic and control experiments were performed simultaneously. After 30 min incubation at $37°C$, filters were removed, fixed and stained with eosin-Y and Giemsa stain. Eosinophils migrated to the lower side of the filter were counted in 10 high-power fields (hpf), and chemotactic and chemokinetic results were expressed as eosinophil counts/hpf.

To determine the effects of a selective PAF antagonist, BN52021 (15), eosinophils were incubated with different concentrations of BN52021 (1×10^{-9}– 1×10^{-4} M) or HBSS for 20 min at $37°C$. Then 2×10^5 eosinophils were applied into the chamber and evaluated for the chemotactic responses toward 1×10^{-7} M of PAF.

To determine the deactivation effects of PAF, eosinophils were incubated with different concentrations of PAF (1×10^{-11} to 1×10^{-7} M) or HBSS for 20 min at $37°C$. After incubation, eosinophils were washed 3 times in HBSS by centrifugation ($400 \times g$ for 10 min at $4°C$) and re-suspended in HBSS. Eosinophils (2×10^{-5}) were applied to evaluate their further chemotactic responses toward 1×10^{-7} M of PAF.

6.2.5 LTC₄ Production from Eosinophils

To determine whether or not chemotactic factors directly induce LTC₄ production from eosinophils, 60 μl of the specified concentration of each chemotactic factor and 240 μl of the eosinophil suspension were applied into a glass tube. Each tube was incubated for 0–60 min at 37°C in a shaking water bath.

To evaluate the effect of cytochalasin B on the chemotactic factor induced LTC_4 production, 240 μl of the eosinophil suspension with or without 5 μg/ml of cytochalasin B was incubated for 10 min at 37°C. The reaction was started by adding 60 μl of each chemotactic factor, and incubated further for 30 min at 37°C.

To determine the maximal and the submaximal effect of A23187, 60 μl of different concentrations of A23187 and 240 μl of the eosinophil suspension were incubated in a tube for 20 min at 37°C.

To determine the modifying effect of each chemotactic factor, PMA or phosphatidylserine on the A23187-induced LTC_4 production, 40 μl of the specified concentration of each chemotactic factor, PMA or phosphatidylserine was placed into a tube. Then 160 μl of the eosinophil suspension was applied and incubated for 30 min. After the incubation, 100 μl of the prewarmed A23187 was mixed into a tube, and incubated further for 20 min.

In all experiments, the reaction was terminated by placing the tubes into an ice-cold water bath and the tubes were subsequently centrifuged at 2000 × g for 3 min at 4°C. Approximately 240 μl of the supernatant was collected and stored at −70°C as a sample. The amount of LTC_4 in a sample was measured within 2 weeks.

6.2.5   Measurement of LTC_4

The quantitation of LTC_4 was performed using a specific LTC_4 radioimmunoassay kit. The actual procedures were performed according to the manufacturer's instruction. The sensitivity of the kit was 10 pg of LTC_4/100 μl of the sample, and the reliable range of the measurement was 25–500 pg/100 μl of the sample. The concentration of LTC_4 which inhibited 50% of the radioligand binding (IC_{50}) obtained from 10 independent experiments was 95.3 ± 5.1 pg/100 μl of the sample. The cross-reactivities of structurally relevant metabolites were negligible (32a), and the presence of chemotactic factors, A23187, cytochalasin B, PMA or phosphatidylserine even at their highest concentration used in this study did not interfere with the measurement of LTC_4. The recovery of exogenously added known amount of LTC_4 in the sample was greater than 90% as previously reported (21).

6.2.6   Statistical Analysis

Results were presented as the mean ± standard error (SEM), unless other-

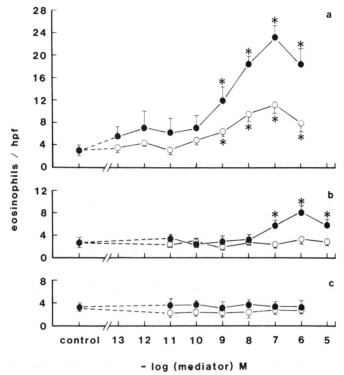

Fig. 1 Eosinophil chemotactic (●) and chemokinetic (○) activities of either PAF (a), ECF-A (b) or LTB₄ (c). Each point represents mean ± SEM of six independent experiments. Asterisk indicates significant (*p* <0.05) activities compared to the control value.

wise stated. The significance of the difference was evaluated using the two-tailed paired t test. The *p* value of <0.05 was considered as a significant difference.

6.3   RESULTS

As shown in Figure 1a, 1×10^{-9} to 1×10^{-6} M of PAF demonstrated both chemotactic and chemokinetic activities for eosinophils. Each chemotactic activity was significantly greater than the chemokinetic activity observed at the same concentration of PAF. Both chemotactic and chemokinetic activities increased in a dose dependent manner, and reached a peak at the concen-

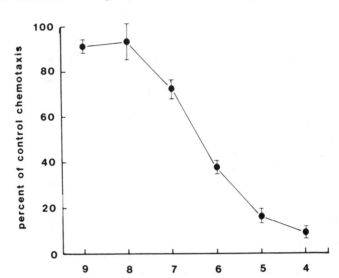

Fig. 2   Dose dependent inhibition of eosinophil responses to 1×10^{-7} M of PAF with BN52021. Eosinophils were preincubated either with a specified concentration of BN52021 or HBSS alone (control) for 20 min at 37°C before chemotactic experiment. Each control response was set at 100%. Each point represents mean ± SEM of six experiments.

tration of 1×10^{-7} M. After reaching the peak, both activities slightly decreased.

As a positive control, ECF-A was used in concentrations of from 1×10^{-11} to 1×10^{-5} M. ECF-A showed the chemotactic activity from the concentration of 1×10^{-7} M to 1×10^{-5} M (Figure 1b). The peak activity of ECF-A was obtained at 1×10^{-6} M. On the other hand, LTB_4 did not show any chemotactic activity for eosinophils from the concentration of 1×10^{-11} to 1×10^{-6} M (Figure 1c).

In order to determine the specificity of PAF-induced chemotaxis, a highly selective PAF antagonist, BN52021, was used. Figure 2 shows the dose-dependent inhibition of PAF-induced eosinophil chemotaxis by BN52021. Significant inhibition was observed at the concentration of 1×10^{-7} M, and the PAF-induced chemotaxis was completely inhibited with 1×10^{-4} M of BN52021. The IC_{50} value of BN52021 calculated was 4.9×10^{-7} M. However, when BN52021 was applied to the upper compartment of the chamber without any pre-incubation period, BN52021 only partially inhibited the chemotaxis, even at the concentration of 1×10^{-4} M (data not shown).

Figure 3 shows the deactivation of eosinophils for further chemotactic responses toward 1×10^{-7} M of PAF after incubation with different concen-

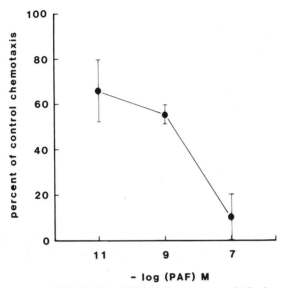

Fig. 3 Deactivation of eosinophil chemotactic responses to PAF after pre-incubation either with a specified concentration of PAF or HBSS alone (control) for 20 min at 37°C. After pre-incubation, eosinophils were washed 3 times in HBSS and applied to further chemotactic responses to 1×10^{-7} M of PAF. Each control response was set at 100%. Each point represents mean ± SEM of five experiments.

trations of PAF. Pre-exposure of eosinophils to 1×10^{-7} M of PAF markedly diminished their chemotactic response ($9.8 \pm 10.1\%$) of control). This effect was observed even at the concentration of 1×10^{-9} M and 1×10^{-11} M of PAF (54.9 ± 3.7 and $65.5 \pm 13.6\%$, respectively).

6.3.1   Direct Effect of Chemotactic Factors on the LTC₄ Production from Eosinophils

In order to evaluate whether or not chemotactic factors directly induce LTC₄ production from eosinophils, eosinophils were incubated with different concentrations of PAF, lyso-PAF, ECF-A and LTB₄ for 30 min at 37°C (Fig. 4). PAF induced LTC₄ production in a dose-dependent manner and 10^{-5} M of PAF induced 0.74 ± 0.08 ng of LTC₄ production/10^6 eosinophils (Fig. 4a). On the other hand, lyso-PAF, an inactive form of PAF, failed to induce LTC₄ production. Different concentrations (10^{-8}–10^{-5} M) of ECF-A (Fig. 4b) and LTB₄ (Fig. 4c) failed to induce LTC₄ production. Using 10^{-6} M of PAF, the time course effect of PAF-induced LTC₄ production was evaluated (Fig. 5).

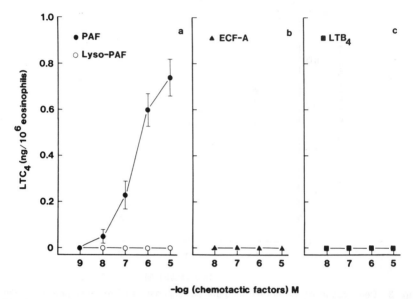

Fig. 4   Direct effect of eosinophil chemotactic factors on the LTC_4 production from eosinophils. Eosinophils were incubated with different concentrations of PAF, lyso-PAF, ECF-A or LTB_4 for 30 min at 37°C. Each point of the PAF-induced LTC_4 production represents the mean ± SEM obtained from 4 independent experiments. Other points (of lyso-PAF, ECF-A or LTB_4) indicate no detectable amount of LTC_4 production observed from each of four independent experiments.

At 5 min incubation of eosinophils, PAF induced LTC_4 production. The amount of LTC_4 produced reached a plateau at 15 min, and remained up to 60 min.

It has been reported that rabbit (33, 34) and human (35) neutrophils respond to PAF only when pre-treated with 5 µg/ml of cytochalasin B. Moreover, Owen et al. (36) reported that human eosinophils produced LTC_4 stimulated by n-formyl-l-methionyl-l-leucyl-L-phenylalanine (fMLP) only when preincubated with 5 µg/ml of cytochalasin B. We therefore evaluated the effect of pre-incubation with 5 µg/ml of cytochalasin B on chemotactic factor-induced LTC_4 production. Cytochalasin B alone did not induce a detectable amount of LTC_4 production from eosinophils, and the pre-incubation of eosinophils with cytochalasin B for 10 min did not alter PAF-induced LTC_4 production (Fig. 6). The incubation of eosinophils with the highest concentration of each chemotactic factor did not affect the viability of eosinophils.

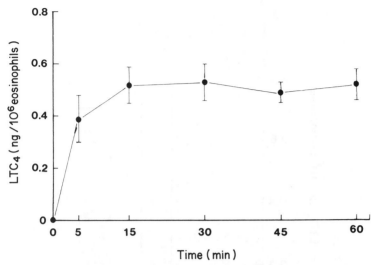

Fig. 5 Time course studies of the PAF-induced LTC₄ production from eosinophils. 10^{-6} M of PAF was added to the eosinophil suspension (time = 0), and incubated for up to 60 min at 37°C. Each point represents the mean ± SEM obtained from 4 independent experiments.

6.3.2 Modifying Effect of Chemotactic Factors on the A23187-induced LTC₄ Production from Eosinophils

Figure 7 shows the concentration-dependent effect of A23187 on LTC₄ production from eosinophils. 1 μg/ml and 5 μg/ml of A23187 induced 5.69 ± 1.00 ng and 46.73 ± 6.47 ng of LTC₄ production/10^6 eosinophils, respectively. The amount of LTC₄ production reached a plateau at 5 μg/ml of A23187. In our further experiments, we chose 1 μg/ml and 5 μg/ml of A23187 as a submaximal and a maximal stimulus, respectively.

We evaluated the effect of pre-incubation of eosinophils with chemotactic factors on the submaximal dose of A23187-induced LTC₄ production. As shown in Figure 8a, pre-incubation with 10^{-6} M and 10^{-5} M of PAF significantly enhanced the A23187-induced LTC₄ production up to 163.9 ± 17.5% ($p < 0.05$) and 279.2 ± 32.9% ($p < 0.01$) of the control, respectively. Lyso-PAF showed a tendency to enhance the A23187-induced LTC₄ production. However, this effect was not statistically significant. The pre-incubation of eosinophils with 10^{-5} M of ECF-A also enhanced the A23187-induced LTC₄ production up to 165.2 ± 21.2% of the control ($p < 0.05$) (Fig. 8b), however LTB₄ failed to enhance or inhibit the LTC₄ production (Fig. 8c).

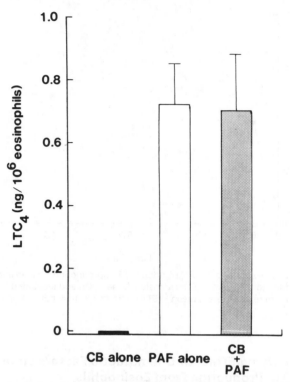

Fig. 6   Effect of cytochalasin B (CB) on the LTC_4 production from eosinophils. To test the direct effect of cytochalasin B, eosinophils were incubated with cytochalasin B (5 μg/ml) for 10 min at 37°C. To test the modifying effect of cytochalasin B on the A23187-induced LTC_4 production, eosinophils were preincubated with cytochalasin B (5 μg/ml) for 10 min at 37°C, and then incubated further with A23187 (1 μg/ml) for 20 min at 37°C. The results indicate the mean ± SEM obtained from four independent experiments.

There was no significant effect of these chemotactic factors if eosinophils were stimulated with the maximal dose of A23187 (data not shown).

6.3.3   Effect of Direct Stimulation of Protein Kinase C by PMA on the A23187-induced LTC_4 Production from Eosinophils

It is known that phorbol myristate acetate (PMA) directly stimulates protein kinase C (37). As shown in Table 1, the stimulation of protein kinase C by different concentrations of PMA alone did not induce LTC_4 production from eosinophils. However, when eosinophils were pre-incubated with PMA, this pre-incubation induced the enhancement effect ($p < 0.05$) on the submaximal

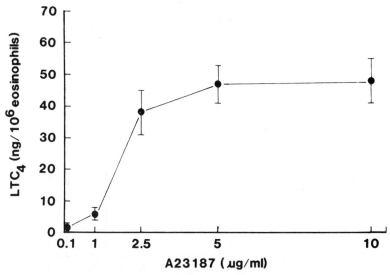

Fig. 7 Dose-dependent effect of calcium ionophore A23187 on the LTC_4 production from eosinophils. Eosinophils were incubated with different concentrations of A23187 for 20 min at 37°C. Each point represents the mean $\pm$ SEM obtained from four independent experiments.

dose of A23187-induced LTC_4 production (179.5 $\pm$ 20.9% of the control at 1 ng/ml of PMA).

6.3.4   Effect of Phosphatidylserine on the A23187-induced LTC_4 Production

We evaluated the non-specific effect of phosphatidylserine as a membrane-derived lipid metabolite on the LTC_4 production. 10^{-5} M of phosphatidylserine did not either induce LTC_4 production or alter the submaximal dose of A23187-induced LTC_4 production from eosinophils (Table 2).

6.4   DISCUSSION

It is well known that ECF-A is a potent eosinophil chemotactic factor, and 10^{-7} M level of ECF-A is chemotactic for eosinophils (38). Our result using ECF-A was comparable, and thus PAF was evaluated to be 100-fold more potent eosinophil chemotactic factor compared with ECF-A (see Fig. 1a, b).

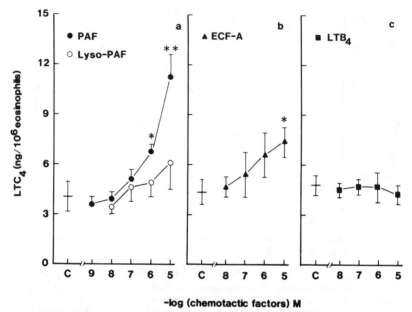

Fig. 8 Modifying effect of eosinophil chemotactic factors on the submaximal dose (1 µg/ml) of A23187-induced LTC$_4$ production from eosinophils. Eosinophils were preincubated with different concentrations of each chemotactic factor for 30 min at 37°C, and then incubated further with A23187 for 20 min at 37°C. Each point represents the mean ±SEM obtained from 9 (for PAF) or 4 (for lyso-PAF, ECF-A or LTB$_4$) independent experiments. * ($p < 0.05$) and ** ($p < 0.01$) indicate a significant difference as compared to each control value.

Since BN52021, a selective PAF antagonist, inhibited PAF-induced eosinophil chemotactic responses in a dose-dependent manner, the PAF-induced eosinophil chemotaxis is through specific PAF receptors. This further suggests the presence of specific PAF receptors on eosinophils.

Only a few studies have reported eosinophil chemotactic responses to PAF (39, 40). In these cases, however, eosinophils were obtained from patients with hypereosinophilia, and they used a lower purity of eosinophils (39) or a mixed granulocyte population (40). Thus, the specificity of PAF action on eosinophils is not clear from these reports.

It has been reported that some of the eosinophils in patients with hypereosinophilia are activated, and usually these activated eosinophils are hypodense eosinophils. Eosinophils obtained, therefore, from patients with hypereosinophilia may not represent those with normal function (41). In this study, we used eosinophils obtained from normal subjects, and these eosinophils were normodense eosinophils (density was greater than 1.085).

Table 1   Effect of protein kinase C activation on the LTC$_4$ production from eosinophils

Pre-incubation	Stimulation	LTC$_4$ production (ng/10^6 eosinophils)
None	PMA 1 ng/ml	Not detectable
None	PMA 10 ng/ml	Not detectable
None	PMA 100 ng/ml	Not detectable
None	A23187 1 μg/ml	4.92 ± 0.22
PMA 1 ng/ml	A23187 1 μg/ml	8.83 ± 1.03*
PMA 10 ng/ml	A23187 1 μg/ml	7.48 ± 1.46
PMA 100 ng/ml	A23187 1 μg/ml	6.66 ± 1.48

Protein kinase C was activated by phorbol myristate acetate (PMA). To determine if the activation of protein kinase C directly induces LTC$_4$ production from eosinophils or not, eosinophils were incubated with PMA for 30 min at 37°C. To test the modifying effect of the activation of protein kinase C on the A23187-induced LTC$_4$ production, eosinophils were preincubated with PMA for 30 min at 37°C, and then incubated further with A23187 (1 μg/ml) for 20 min at 37°C. The amount of LTC$_4$ was presented as the mean ± SEM obtained from four independent experiments.
* indicates the statistical difference ($p < 0.05$) as compared to the control.

ECF-A has been reported to induce eosinophil deactivation for further chemotactic responses (38). In order to determine whether or not PAF possesses the same characteristic, we incubated eosinophils with different concentrations of PAF, washed 3 times and applied them to the chemotactic chambers containing 1×10^{-7} M of PAF. Pre-incubation of eosinophils with 1×10^{-7} M of PAF significantly inhibited the further chemotactic responses to 1×10^{-7} M of PAF. The precise mechanism of deactivation is still unclear.

We did not observe any chemotactic responses of eosinophils toward a wide concentration range of LTB$_4$. Our findings contrast with those observed

Table 2   Effect of phosphatidylserine (PS) on the LTC$_4$ production from eosinophils

Pre-incubation	Stimulation	LTC$_4$ production (ng/10^6 eosinophils)
None	PS 10^{-5} M	Not detectable
None	A23187 1 μg/ml	4.69 ± 0.45
PS 10^{-5} M	A23187 1 μg/ml	5.38 ± 1.23

To test if phosphatidylserine (PS) directly induces LTC$_4$ production from eosinophils or not, eosinophils were incubated with 10^{-5} M of phosphatidylserine for 30 min at 37°C. To test the modifying effect of phosphatidylserine on the A23187-induced LTC$_4$ production, eosinophils were pre-incubated with 10^{-5} M of phosphatidylserine for 30 min at 37°C, and then incubated further with A23187 for 20 min at 37°C. The amount of LTC$_4$ produced was presented at the mean ± SEM obtained from four independent experiments.

by Czarnetzki *et al.* (40). Although the reason for this discrepancy is not very clear, the purity of the eosinophils used in the study could be responsible for such controversy. It should be pointed out that LTB_4 induces calcium increase in neutrophils (42) and PAF formation requires calcium increase in cells (43). Thus using eosinophils with a high percentage of neutrophil contamination, LTB_4 may trigger the release of chemical mediators from neutrophils; these chemical mediators, including PAF, might then cause eosinophil activation. In our system, we have used highly purified eosinophils to avoid such problems.

Our data provide the evidence that PAF attracts normal eosinophils and this activity is the strongest so far reported. PAF may therefore play an important role in the pathogenesis of bronchial asthma.

Eosinophils may contribute to the pathogenesis of bronchial asthma both by the injurious effect of the airway tract, and by the production of LTC_4. In this study, however, we have focused on the LTC_4 production as a marker of eosinophil functions.

It is well known that LTC_4 is enzymatically converted to LTD_4 by γ-glutamyl transpeptidase and, finally, to LTE_4. Furthermore, when stimulated by calcium ionophore (44) and by specific IgE antibodies (45), eosinophils produce eosinophil peroxidase. Eosinophil peroxidase, in the presence of H_2O_2 and halides, inactivates LTC_4 activity (44), and metabolizes LTC_4 to 6-trans LTB_4 (19). Such biodegradation therefore makes it very difficult to assess accurately the amount of LTC_4, unless the assay is carried out under conditions that prevent such bioconversion and a measurement method is used which is highly specific for LTC_4. It has been reported that the serine–borate complex inhibits γ-glutamyl transpeptidase activity (46, 47), and 1-serine prevents the oxidative metabolism of LTC_4 to 6-trans LTB_4 (19). We have used the serine–borate complex not only in the measurement processes but in the processes of LTC_4 production. Furthermore, a highly specific and sensitive LTC_4 radioimmunoassay kit enabled us to measure LTC_4 more accurately without any significant cross-reactivities to other arachidonic acid metabolites.

Within the 30 min incubation, PAF directly induced LTC_4 production from eosinophils in a dose-dependent manner. On the other hand, lyso-PAF, ECF-A and LTB_4 failed to induce a detectable amount of LTC_4 production from eosinophils within the tested concentration. It has been reported that PAF induces LTC_4 production from isolated buffer-perfused rat lung (48), rat heart (49) and rat small intestine (50). In all cases, however, the cell source of LTC_4 was quite unknown. In human studies, it has been reported that lung tissue (51) and neutrophils (52) possess specific PAF-binding sites, and PAF induces LTB_4 production from neutrophils (53). Bruijnzeel *et al.* (54)

reported that 10^{-5} M of PAF induces LTC_4 production from human eosinophils in the presence of exogenously added glutathione, which works as a cofactor for the formation of LTC_4 from LTA_4 (3). Our data here, in the absence of exogenously added glutathione, virtually indicated PAF-induced LTC_4 production from human eosinophils, although it is not clear whether or not this amount of LTC_4 production (less than 1 $ng/10^6$ eosinophils) is biologically significant *in vivo*. Neither is it well established whether the induction of LTC_4 production from eosinophils by chemotactic factors is unique to PAF.

The requirement of cytochalasin B for the induction of cell functions is complicated and controversial. Owen *et al.* (36) speculated that the requirement for pre-incubation with cytochalasin B for fMLP to elicit LT generation may relate to the ability of cytochalasin B to up-regulate the reversible binding of fMLP. PAF-induced arachidonic acid release from rabbit neutrophils (33), rabbit neutrophil degranulation (34) and protein kinase C mobilization in human neutrophils (35) require the presence of cytochalasin B. On the other hand, PAF-induced phosphatidic acid formation and serotonin release from rabbit platelets (55), and LTB_4 production from human neutrophils (53) did not require the presence of cytochalasin B. Moreover, the presence of cytochalasin B inhibited PAF-induced human monocyte aggregation (56). The fMLP-induced LTC_4 production from human eosinophils required the presence of cytochalasin B (36), but the presence of cytochalasin B did not alter the fMLP-induced human monocyte aggregation (56). In our experiment, the pre-incubation of eosinophils with 5 $\mu g/ml$ of cytochalasin B (the same concentration as reported by others (33–36, 56)) did not alter 10^{-5} M of PAF-induced LTC_4 production from eosinophils.

The pre-incubation of eosinophils with 10^{-5} M and 10^{-6} M of PAF, and with 10^{-5} M of ECF-A significantly enhanced the LTC_4 production induced by the submaximal dose (1 $\mu g/ml$) of A23187. On the other hand, the preincubation of eosinophils with LTB_4 did not alter the LTC_4 production. When stimulated by the maximal dose (5 $\mu g/ml$) of A23187, these preincubations with PAF and ECF-A did not alter the LTC_4 production. These enhancement effects seem to be synergistic but not just additive, because PAF alone induced less than 1 ng of LTC_4 production$/10^6$ eosinophils and ECF-A alone did not induce detectable amount of LTC_4 production. It has been reported that the inhalation of PAF induces non-specific airway reactivity in guinea-pigs (57), rats (58), rhesus monkeys (59), dogs (60) and humans (61). The precise mechanism of the induction of the airway hyperreactivity is unclear. However, the enhancement effect of the LTC_4 production from eosinophils by PAF could be a part of the mechanisms. Although we did not present any data here, PAF-induced enhancement effect could also be true for the release of eosinophil granules which induce an injurious effect on airways, thereby increasing airway reactivity.

It should be noted that not only PAF but also ECF-A enhanced LTC_4 production from eosinophils. Recombinant granulocyte–macrophage colony stimulating factor (GM-CSF) (62) and monokines (63) have been reported to enhance A23187-induced LTC_4 production from eosinophils. Because of the short duration (within 60 min) of the incubation period that produced maximum enhancement, both reports concluded that protein synthesis was not required for their effects. In our experiment, PAF and ECF-A induced their effects at 30 min. These effects do not, therefore, seem to require protein synthesis.

It has been reported that ECF-A induces the increases of the complement- and the IgG-receptor-mediated rosette formation of eosinophils (64, 65). These studies of heterologous up-regulation of the receptor number by ECF-A could be a part of the mechanisms of the enhancement of the receptor-mediated LTC_4 production. However, very importantly, as we presented in this study, PAF and ECF-A enhanced the A23187-induced LTC_4 production, which is not receptor-mediated. This suggests the involvement of a mechanism which is regulated beyond the receptor.

It is known that chemotactic peptides and PAF exert their effects on the cell calcium ion by interacting with surface receptors (66) and, at least in neutrophils, these chemotactic receptors transduce their signals through the activation of phospholipase C (67). The activation of phospholipase C activates phosphatidylinositol turnover, and resulting diacylglycerol activates protein kinase C (68). In general, it is believed that the induction of the cell functions by chemotactic factors require both the activation of protein kinase C and the increase of the intracellular calcium concentration (68). In this study, the direct activation of protein kinase C by PMA alone did not induce LTC_4 production from eosinophils; however, the pre-incubation of eosinophils with 1 ng/ml of PMA significantly enhanced the LTC_4 production induced by the submaximal dose of A23187. A schematic diagram depicting the interaction of A23187 and PMA on protein kinase C and LTC_4 production is shown in Figure 9. The concentrations of PMA used in this study (1–100 ng/ml) are known to activate protein kinase C and induce the mobilization of protein kinase C from cytosol to cell membrane (69). In fact, it has been reported that calcium mobilization and protein kinase C activation are synergistically involved in the release of serotonin from platelets (70) and, in many types of cells, it is suggested that the synergism may be due to the combined effects of calcium and the activation of protein kinase C (66). This could be a part of the mechanisms of PAF- and ECF-A-induced enhancement of the LTC_4 production from eosinophils. Another possibility, especially for the PAF-induced

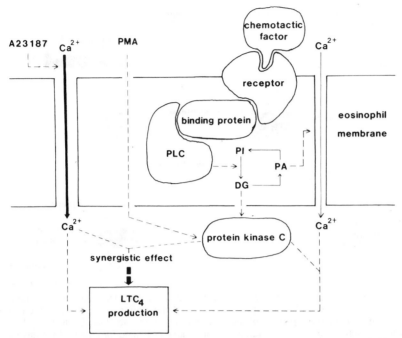

Fig. 9 Schematic diagram depicting the interaction of A23187 and PMA on protein kinase C and LTC₄ production. Chemotactic peptides and PAF interact with cell surface receptors and transduce their signals through activation of phospholipase C (PLC). The activation of phospholipase C activates phosphatidylinositol (PI) turnover, and resulting diacylglycerol (DG) activates protein kinase C. The pre-incubation of eosinophils with PMA significantly enhanced the LTC₄ production induced by the submaximal dose of A23187.

enhancement of LTC$_4$ production, is that a very high concentration of membrane lipid related component, re-inserted into the cell membrane, and this might alter the membrane permeability. However, this is unlikely because the pre-incubation of eosinophils with 10^{-5} M of phosphatidylserine or LTB$_4$ did not alter the A23187-induced LTC$_4$ production.

We propose finally to present a hypothetical model of the activation of eosinophils by chemotactic factors (Fig. 10). As previously reported (30), PAF induced eosinophil chemotaxis from 10^{-9} M level and the peak activity was obtained at 10^{-7} M. ECF-A induced eosinophil chemotaxis from 10^{-7} M level and the peak activity was at 10^{-6} M. In both cases, higher concentrations of chemotactic factors induced less chemotaxis than their optimal concentrations. These observations were quite similar to those reported by Wardlaw et al. (29). The less activity at higher concentration of the chemotactic factor seems to be due to the rapid induction of the deactivation of eosi-

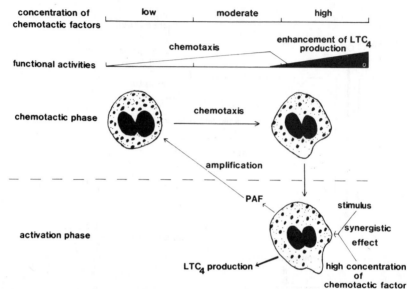

Fig. 10   A hypothetical model of the activation of eosinophils by eosinophil chemotactic factors. Initially, eosinophils are attracted to the inflammatory site according to the low to moderate concentration gradient of the chemotactic factor. And at moderate-to-high concentration of the chemotactic factor, eosinophils are deactivated for further chemotaxis and stay as potential effector cells (chemotactic phase). Then eosinophils are activated synergistically by the stimulus which increases intracellular calcium concentration, and by the presence of high concentration of the chemotactic factor activated eosinophils are induced to produce enhanced LTC_4 production or possibly other functions as effector cells (activation phase). PAF produced from activated eosinophils may further amplify and induce the vicious cycle of the inflammation.

nophils for further chemotaxis. In this study, however, 10^{-6} M and 10^{-5} M of PAF, and 10^{-5} M of ECF-A (only at high concentrations of the chemotactic factors) induced the enhancement of the LTC_4 production. Although the experimental conditions were different, these two observations (chemotaxis and enhancement of LTC_4 production) are clearly dose-dependent phenomena. Furthermore, eosinophils might contain low- and high-affinity receptors for chemotactic factors: one of them may mediate chemotaxis, and the activation of the other receptor produce LTC_4 generation. A similar phenomenon has been observed for LTB_4 receptors in neutrophils, where binding of LTB_4 to low-affinity receptors results in neutrophil degranulation and binding to high affinity receptors promotes aggregation and chemotaxis of neutrophils (71).

Taken together with these observations, initially according to the concentration gradient of the chemotactic factor, eosinophils are attracted by the low-to-moderate concentration of the chemotactic factor. However, at moderate-to-high concentration of the chemotactic factor, eosinophils are deactivated for further chemotaxis and stay at the inflammatory site as potential effector cells (chemotactic phase). At the inflammatory site, eosinophils are then activated synergistically by the stimulus that increases intracellular calcium concentration and by the presence of high concentration of the chemotactic factor activated eosinophils are induced to produce enhanced LTC_4 production or possibly other functions as effector cells (activation phase). When activated, eosinophils produce PAF (72), and this may further amplify and induce the vicious cycle of the inflammation. Although this model may not represent all of the inflammatory processes where eosinophils play an important role, we believe that this hypothetical model explains at least a part of the mechanisms of eosinophil accumulation and activation at the inflammatory site.

Acknowledgements

We would like to thank Dr J. Rokach for synethetic LTB_4. Also, we would like to thank Mrs Debra A. Weber for the recruitment and scheduling of patients, and Mrs Rosemary Batts for the preparation of the manuscript. This work was supported in part by the James M. Keck Faculty Development Award of the Health Future Foundation to D. K. Agrawal.

REFERENCES

1. Nadel, J. A. and Sheppard, D. (1985). Mechanisms of bronchial hyperreactivity in asthma. In "Bronchial Asthma. Mechanisms and Therapeutics" (Eds E. B. Weiss, M. S. Segal and M. Stein), 30–36. Little, Brown, Boston.
2. Boushey, H. A. and Holtzman, M. J. (1985). Experimental airway inflammation and hyperreactivity. Searching for cells and mediators. Am. Rev. Respir. Dis. 131, 312–313.
3. Henderson, W. J. Jr. (1987). Lipid-described and other chemical mediators of inflammation in the lung. J. Allergy Clin. Immunol. 79, 543–553.
4. Weiss, J. W., Drazen, J. M., Coles, N., McFadden, E. R. Jr., Weller, P. F., Corey, E. J., Lewis, R. A. and Austen, K. F. (1982). Bronchoconstrictor effects of leukotriene C in humans. Science 21, 196–198.
5. Smith, L. J., Greenberger, P. A., Patterson, R., Krell, R. D. and Bernstein, P. R. (1985). The effect of inhaled leukotriene D_4 in humans. Am. Rev. Respir. Dis. 131, 368–372.
6. Davidson, A. B., Lee, T. H., Scanlon, P. D., Solway, J., McFadden, E. R. Jr., Ingram, R. H. Jr., Corey, E. J., Austen, K. F. and Drazen, J. M. (1987). Bronchoconstrictor effects of leukotriene E_4 in normal and asthmatic subjects. Am. Rev. Respir. Dis. 135, 333–337.

7. Benveniste, J., Henson, P. M. and Cochrane, C. G. (1972). *J. Exp. Med.* **136**, 1356–1377.
8. Chignard, M., LeCouedic, J. P., Vargaftig, B. B. and Benveniste, J. (1980). *Br. J. Haematol.* **46**, 455–464.
9. Betz, S. J., Lotner, G. Z. and Henson, P. M. (1980). *J. Immunol.* **125**, 2756–2763.
10. Mencia-Huerta, J. M. and Benveniste, J. (1979). *Eur. J. Immunol.* **9**, 409–415.
11. Lee, T-C., Lenihan, D. J., Malone, B., Roddy, L. L. and Wasserman, S. I. (1984). *J. Biol. Chemist.* **259**, 5526–5530.
12. Vargaftig, B. B., Chigard, M., Benveniste, J., Lefort, J. and Wal, F. (1981). *Ann. N Y Acad. Sci.* **370**, 119–137.
13. Archer, C. B., Page, C. P., Morley, J. and MacDonald, D. M. (1985). *Br. J. Dermatol.* **112**, 285–290.
14. Lellouch-Tubiana, A., Lefort, J., Pirotzky, E., Vargaftig, B. B. and Pfister, A. (1985). *Br. J. Exp. Path.* **66**, 345–355.
15. Morley, J., Page, C. P. and Paul, W. (1983). *Br. J. Pharmac.* **80**, 503–509.
16. Goetzl, E. J., Derian, C. K., Tauber, A. I. and Valone, F. H. (1980). *Biochem. Biophys, Res. Commun.* **94**, 881–888.
17. Kay, A. B. (1985). Eosinophils and neutrophils in the pathogenesis of asthma. *In* "Bronchial Asthma. Mechanisms and Therapeutics" (Eds E. B. Weiss, M. S. Segal and M. Stein), 255–265. Little, Brown, Boston.
18. Frigas, E. and Gleich, G. J. (1986). The eosinophil and the pathophysiology of asthma. *J. Allergy Clin. Immunol.* **77**, 527–537.
19. Weller, P. F., Lee, C. W., Foster, D. W., Corey, E. J., Austen, K. F. and Lewis, R.A. (1983). Generation and metabolism of 5-lipoxygenase pathway leukotrienes by human eosinophils: Predominant production of leukotriene C_4. *Proc. Natl. Acad. Sci. USA.* **80**, 7626–7630.
20. Shaw, R.J., Cromwell, O. and Kay, A. B. (1984). Preferential generation of leukotriene C_4 by human eosinophils. *Clin. Exp. Med.* **56**, 716–722.
21. Tamura, N., Agrawal, D. K. and Townley, R. G. (1987). A specific radioreceptor assay for leukotriene C_4 and the measurement of calcium ionophore-induced leukotriene C_4 production from human leukocytes. *J. Pharmacol. Methods* **18**, 327–333.
22. Shaw, R. J., Walsh, G. M., Cromwell, O., Moqbel, R., Spray, C. J. F. and Kay, A. B. (1985). Activated human eosinophils generate SRS-A leukotrienes following IgG-dependent stimulation. *Nature* **316**, 150–152.
23. Wang, S. R., Yang, C. M., Wang, S. S. M., Han, S. H. and Chiang, B. N. (1986). Enhancement of A23187-induced production of the slow-reacting substance on peripheral leukocytes from subjects with asthma. *J. Allergy Clin. Immunol.* **77**, 465–471.
24. Kauffman, H. F., van der Belt, B., DeMonchy, J. G. R., Boelens, H., Koeter, G. H. and de Vries, K. (1987). Leukotriene C_4 production by normal-density and low-density eosinophils of atopic individuals and other patients with eosinophila. *J. Allergy Clin. Immunol.* **79**, 611–619.
25. Fukuda, T., Dunnette, S. L., Reed, C. E., Ackerman, S. J., Peters, M. S. and Gleich, G. J. (1985). Increased numbers of hypodense eosinophils in the blood of patients with bronchial asthma. *Am. Rev. Respir. Dis.* **132**, 981–985.
26. De Monchy, J. G. R., Kauffman, H. F., Venge, P., Koeter, G. H., Jansen, H. M., Sluiter, H. J. and de Vries, K. (1985). Bronchoalveolar eosinophilia during allergen-induced late asthmatic reactions. *Am. Rev. Respir. Dis.* **131** 373–376.

27. Metzger, W. J., Richerson, H. B. and Wasserman, S.I. (1986). Generation and partial characterization of eosinophil chemotactic activity during early and late-phase asthmatic response. *J. Allergy Clin. Immunol.* **78**, 282–290.
28. Cohen, S. G. and Ottesen, E. A. (1983). The eosinophil, eosinophilia, and eosinophil-related disorders. *In* "Allergy. Principles and Practice" (Eds E. Middleton, Jr., C. H. Reed and E. F. Ellis), 701–769. C. V. Mosby, St. Louis.
29. Wardlaw, A. J., Moqbel, R., Cromwell, O. and Kay, A. B. (1986). Platelet-activating factor. A potent chemotactic and chemokinetic factor for human eosinophils. *J. Clin. Invest.* **78**, 1701–1706.
30. Tamura, N., Agrawal, D. K., Suliaman, F. A. and Townley, R. G. (1987). Effects of platelet-activating factor on the chemotaxis of normodense eosinophils from normal subjects. *Biochem. Biophys. Res. Commun.* **142**, 638–644.
31. Goetzl, E. J. and Austen, K. F. (1976). Structural determinants of the eosinophil chemotactic activity of the acidic tetrapeptides of eosinophil chemotactic factor of anaphylaxis. *J. Exp. Med.* **144**, 1424–1437.
32. Randolph, T. G. (1944). Blood studies in allergy. I. The direct counting chamber determination of eosinophils by propylene glycol aqueous stains. *J. Allergy* **15**, 89–96.
32a. Wynalda, M. A., Brashler, J. R., Bach, M. K., Morton, D. R. and Fitzpatrick, F. A. (1984). Determination of leukotriene C_4 by radioimmunoassay with a specific antiserum generated from a synthetic hapten mimic. *Anal. Chem.* **56**, 1862–1865.
33. Chilton, F. H., O'Flaherty, J. T., Walsh, C. E., Thomas, M. J., Wykle, R. L., DeChatelet, L. R. and Waite, B. M. (1982). Platelet activating factor. Stimulation of the lipoxygenase pathway in polymorphonuclear leukocytes by 1-*o*-alkyl-2-*o*-acetyl-*sn*-glycero-3-phosphocholine. *J. Biol. Chem.* **257**, 5402–5407.
34. O'Flaherty, J. T., Swendsen, C. L., Lees, C. J. and McCall, C. E. (1981). Role of extracellular calcium in neutrophil degranulation responses to 1-*o*-alkyl-2-*o*-acetyl-*sn*-glycero-3-phosphocholine. *Am. J. Pathol.* **105**, 107–113.
35. O'Flaherty, J. T. and Nishihara, J. (1987). Arachidonate metabolites, platelet-activating factor, and the mobilization of protein kinase C in human polymorphonuclear neutrophils. *J. Immunol.* **138**, 1889–1895.
36. Owen, W. F. Jr., Soberman, R. J., Yoshimoto, T., Sheffer, A. L. Lewis, R. A. and Austen, K. F. (1987). Synthesis and release of leukotriene C_4 by human eosinophils. *J. Immunol.* **138**, 532–538.
37. Castagna, M., Takai, Y., Kaibuchi, K., Sano, K., Kikkawa, U. and Nishizuka, Y. (1982). Direct activation of calcium-activated, phospholipid-dependent protein kinase by tumor-promoting phorbol esters. *J. Biol. Chem.* **257**, 7847–7851.
38. Goetzl, E. J. and Austen, K. F. (1975). *Proc. Natl. Acad. Sci. USA* **72**, 4123–4128.
39. Wardlaw, A. J. and Kay, A. B. (1986). *J. Allergy Clin. Immunol.* (abstr.) **77**, 464.
40. Czarnetzki, B. M. and Rosenbach, T. (1986). Chemotaxis of human neutrophils and eosinophils towards leukotriene B_4 and its 20-*w*-oxidation products *in vitro*. *Prostaglandins* **31**, 851–858.
41. Winqvist, I., Olofsson, T., Olsson, I., Persson, A-M. and Hallberg, T. (1982). *Immunology* **47**, 531–539.
42. Goldman, D. W., Gifford, L. A., Olson, D. M. and Goetzl, E. J. (1985). *J. Immunol.* **135**, 525–530.
43. Anderson, W. H. (1985). *In* "Bronchial Asthma" (Eds. E. B. Weiss, M. S. Segal and M. Stein), 57–58. Little, Brown, Boston.

44. Henderson, W. R., Jorg, A. and Klebanoff, S. J. (1982). Eosinophil peroxidase-mediated inactivation of leukotrienes B_4, C_4, and D_4. *J. Immunol.* **128**, 2609–2613.
45. Khalife, J., Capron, M., Cesbron, J-Y., Tai, P-C., Taelman, H., Prin, L. and Capron, A. (1986). Role of specific IgE antibodies in peroxidase (EPO) release from human eosinophils. *J. Immunol.* **137**, 1659–1664.
46. Tate, S. S. and Meister, A. (1978). Serine-borate complex as a transition-state inhibitor of γ-glutamyl transpeptidase. *Proc. Natl. Acad. Sci. USA.* **75**, 4806–4809.
47. Cheng, J. B. and Townley, R. G. (1984). Effect of the serine–borate complex on the relative ability of leukotriene C_4, D_4 and E_4 to inhibit lung and brain $[^3H]$leukotriene D_4 and $[^3H]$leukotriene C_4 binding: Demonstration of the agonists' potency order for leukotriene D_4 and leukotriene C_4 receptors. *Biochem. Biophys. Res. Commun.* **119**, 612–617.
48. Voelkel, N. F., Worthen, S., Reeves, J. T., Henson, P. M. and Murphy, R. C. (1982). Nonimmunological production of leukotrienes induced by platelet-activating factor. *Science* **218**, 286–288.
49. Piper, P. J. and Stewart, A. G. (1986). Coronary vasoconstriction in the rat, isolated perfused heart induced by platelet-activating factor is mediated by leukotriene C_4. *Br. J. Pharmac.* **88**, 595–605.
50. Hsueh, W., Gonzalez-Crussi, F. and Arroyave, J. L. (1986). Release of leukotriene C_4 by isolated, perfused rat small intestine in response to platelet-activating factor. *J. Clin. Invest.* **78**, 108–114.
51. Hwang, S-B., Lam, M-H. and Shen, T. Y. (1985). Specific binding sites for platelet activating factor in human lung tissues. *Biochem. Biophys. Res. Commun.* **128**, 972–979.
52. O'Flaherty, J. T., Surles, J. R., Redman, J., Jacobson, D., Piantadosi C., and Wykle, R. L. (1986). Binding and metabolism and platelet-activating factor by human neutrophils. *J. Clin. Invest.* **78**, 381–388.
53. Lin, A. H., Morton, D. R. and Gorman, R. R. (1982). Acetyl glyceryl ether phosphorylcholine stimulates leukotriene B_4 synthesis in human polymorphonuclear leukocytes. *J. Clin. Invest.* **70**, 1058–1065.
54. Bruijnzeel. P. L. B., Koenderman, L., Kok, P. T. M., Hameling, M. L. and Verhagen, J. (1986). Platelet-activating factor (PAF-acether) induced leukotriene C_4 formation and luminol dependent chemiluminescence by human eosinophils. *Pharmac. Res. Commun.* **18**, 61–70 (suppl.).
55. Shukla, S. D. and Hanahan, D. J. (1984). Acetylglyceryl ether phosphorylcholine (AGEPC; platelet-activating factor)-induced stimulation of rabbit platelets: Correlation between phosphatidic acid level, $^{45}Ca^{2+}$ uptake, and $[^3H]$serotonin secretion. *Arch. Biochem. Biophys.* **232**, 458–466.
56. Yasaka, T., Boxer, L. A. and Baehner, R. L. (1982). Monocyte aggregation and superoxide anion release in response to formyl-methionyl-leucyl-phenylalanine (FMLP) and platelet-activating factor (PAF). *J. Immunol.* **128**, 1939–1944.
57. Mazzoni, L., Morley, J., Page, C. P. and Sanjar, S., (1985). Induction of airway hyperreactivity by platelet activating factor in the guinea-pig. *J. Physiol.* **365**, 107p (suppl.).
58. Chand, N., Mahoney, T. P., Diamantis, W. and Sofia, R.D. (1986). The amplification role of platelet activating factor (PAF), other chemical mediators and antigen in the induction of airway hyperreactivity to cold. *Eur. J. Pharmacol.* **123**, 315–317.
59. Patterson, R., Bernstein, P. R., Harris K. E. and Krell, R. D. (1984) Airway re-

sponses to sequential challenges with platelet-activating factor and leukotriene D_4 in rhesus monkeys. *J. Lab. Clin. Med.* **104**, 340–345.

60. Chung, K. F. Aizawa, H., Leikauf, G. D., Ueki, I. F., Evans, T. W. and Nadel, J. A. (1986). Airway hyperresponsiveness induced by platelet-activating factor: Role of thromboxane generation. *J. Pharmacol. Exp. Ther.* **236**, 580–584.

61. Cuss, F. M., Dixon, C. M. S. and Barnes, P. J. (1986). Effects of inhaled platelet activating factor on pulmonary function and bronchial responsiveness in man. *Lancet* **II**, 189–192.

62. Silberstein, D. S., Owen, W. F., Gasson, J. C., DiPersio, J. F., Golde, D. W., Bina, J. C., Soberman, R., Austen, K. F. and David, J. R. (1986). Enhancement of human eosinophil cytotoxicity and leukotriene synthesis by biosynthetic (recombinant) granulocyte-macrophage colony-stimulating factor. *J. Immunol.* **137**, 3290–3294.

63. Dessein, A.J., Lee, T. H., Elasas, P., Ravelese, J. III, Silberstein, D., David, J. R., Austen, K. F. and Lewis, R. A. (1986). Enhancement by monokines of leukotriene generation by human eosinophils and neutrophils stimulated with calcium ionophore A23187. *J. Immunol.* **136**, 3829–3838.

64. Anwar, A. R. E. and Kay, A. B. (1978). Enhancement of human eosinophil complement receptors by pharmacological mediators. *J. Immunol.* **121**, 1245–1250.

65. Capron, M., Capron, A., Goetzl, E. J. and Austen, K. F. (1981). Tetrapeptides of the eosinophil chemotactic factor of anaphylaxis (ECF-A) enhance eosinophil Fc receptor. *Nature* **289**, 71–73.

66. Exton, J. H. (1985). Role of calcium and phosphoinositides in the action of certain hormones and neurotransmitters. *J. Clin. Invest.* **75**, 1753–1757.

67. Snyderman, R., Smith, C. D. and Verghese, M. W. (1986). Model for leukocyte regulation by chemoattractant receptors: Roles of a guanine nucleotide regulatory protein and polyphosphoinositide metabolism. *J. Leukocyte Biol.* **40**, 785–800.

68. Berridge, M. J. (1985). Calcium-mobilizing receptors. Membrane phosphoinositides and signal transduction. *In* "Calcium in Biological Systems" (Eds R. P. Rubin, G. B. Weiss and J. W. Putney Jr.), 37–44. Plenum Press, New York.

69. Nagao, S., Nagata, K., Kohmura, Y., Ishizuka, T. and Nozawa, Y. (1987). Redistribution of phospholipid/Ca^{2+}-dependent protein kinase in mast cells activated by various agonists. *Biochem. Biophys. Res. Commun.* **142**, 645–653.

70. Kaibuchi, K., Sano, K., Hoshijima, M., Takai, Y., Nishizuka, Y. (1982). Phosphatidylinositol turnover in platelet activation; Calcium mobilization and protein phosphorylation. *Cell Calcium* **3**, 323–335.

71. Goldman, D. W. and Goetzl, E. J. (1984). Heterogeneity of human polymorphonuclear leukocyte receptors for leukotriene B_4. *J. Exp. Med.* **159**, 1027–1041.

72. Lee, T-C., Lenihan, D. J., Malone, B., Roddy, L. L. and Wasserman, S. I. (1984). Increased biosynthesis of platelet-activating factor in activated human eosinophils. *J. Biol. Chem.* **259**, 5526–5530.

DISCUSSION

Makino (Chairman)

Vadas: We are talking about chemotactic agents, so I shall just put the converse story as subject for discussion. If you pretreat a population of neutrophils with GM-CSF and then ask them to move in a chemotactic gradient. They are substantially inhibited in their movement when compared with untreated neutrophils. Agents that activate these cells also inhibit their capacity to move in a chemotactic gradient. This could be interpreted as a stand-and-fight response invoked in neutrophils by cytokines and we have preliminary evidence that it's the same in eosinophils.

Wasserman: I'd like to direct a question to any of the people who have worked with eosinophil chemotaxis and have looked at the various inhibitors of PAF. It's clear that the inhibitors all inhibit PAF induced chemotaxis. Has anyone looked at the PAF inhibitors for their ability to inhibit any other form of eosinophil movement, for example C5a induced eosinophil directed movement or the minor degree of chemotaxis seen with ECF-A? The interpretation that PAF is a responsible agent requires that it be demonstrated that these PAF inhibitors are not only specific but selective.

Kay: We have tested a whole range of chemotactic factors including C5a, fMLP, LTB$_4$, a purified mononuclear cell derived chemotactic factor from a PHA supernatant and none of them was inhibited by this gingkolide derived compound.

Wasserman: Have you looked at anaphylactic diffusate or anaphylactic supernatant to see if the PAF compound inhibited most of the activity seen there?

Fukuda: We tested the factor CV 3988 which is a selective PAF antagonist on eosinophil chemotaxis induced by zymosan-activated serum and fMLP. CV 3988 did not inhibit eosinophil chemotaxis to these stimuli, so I think that it is specific for PAF.

Wasserman: It seems to be a possibility, however, that the availability of a PAF receptor on eosinophils is important for chemotaxis. Any signals for eosinophil chemotaxis may interact eventually with that receptor. So in interpreting the anaphylactic diffusate, the story remains confusing.

Vargaftig: As I mentioned earlier, the two PAF antagonists, the ginkolyde and WEB 2086, the Boehringer–Ingelheim compound, not only block PAF induced chemotaxis of eosinophils *in vivo*, 6–24 hours after PAF injection, but also antigen induced chemotaxis. The second point is interesting, possibly other agonists should be tested. I was interested that CV 3988 did not only block PAF induced chemotaxis but also chemotaxis induced by the interaction with allergen. Now, I would like to give a word of caution. We have unpublished data that if you inject PAF into an isolated guinea-pig lung, you have some effects—thromboxane release for instance—and this is blocked by all PAF antagonists. So you are satisfied that an anti-PAF blocks PAF, which is not a big surprise. If you remove the lung from a sensitized animal, provided it is an actively sensitized animal, the threshold for PAF is lowered about a 1000 times and when you inject the lower doses of PAF, you have 50% bronchoconstriction. Now, under these conditions, when you test the PAF antagonists, the same antagonists which block PAF in naive lungs, they do not block PAF anymore. The gingkolide derivative and WEB 2086 were anti-PAF in the naive lung, but not anti-PAF in the sensitized lung. However, when we tested PAF antagonists with a glycerol backbone, CV 3988, ROCHE 19-3704, the new TAKEDA compound, plus two other phospholipids provided by Jean-Jaques Godfrid from Paris University, they were effective against PAF on the naive lung as well as on the sensitized lung, new cells are offering different PAF receptors. Other PAF antagonists should be checked, and maybe eosinophils from sensitized patients or animals would have a differential pharmacology according to the PAF antagonist used.

Colditz: I'd like to make a couple of cautionary comments about chemotaxis and its role in the accumulation of leukocytes in vivo. The first relates to work that Dr Boris Vargaftig mentioned, where intravenous injection of PAF in guinea-pigs caused accumulation of eosinophils in the lung. We have similar results from our own lab where intraperitoneal or subcutaneous injection of PAF causes accumulation of eosinophils in the lung as assessed by bronchoalveolar lavage. This obviously contradicts the idea of a chemotactic mechanism recruiting eosinophils out of blood vessels and into the lung, because the highest concentration of PAF, when it is available for its very short half-life, would be within the blood vessel, not outside. The second comment relates to the activity of chemotactic factors in skin and their ability to recruit neutrophils into inflammatory sites. This work was done in rabbits, and we found that chemotactic factors, leukotriene B_4, PAF, fMLP and agents like endotoxin or whole zymosan particles, when injected into skin sites, caused stimulus specific desensitization of those skin sites. When the sites were restimulated with the same agent (e.g. fMLP) they were desensitized to the inflammatory effect of that agent and no further neutrophils would enter the sites, but when sites were re-stimulated with a separate chemotactic factor, there was a normal migration of neutrophils into that skin site. This result indicates that diffusion of a chemotactic factor from an extravascular space across the blood vessel wall isn't a sufficient stimulus to cause migration of cells out of the blood vessel and into the tissue site. This migration of cells is much more complex than the simple notion of chemotaxis.

Townley: Studies that Dr Vargaftig has mentioned and also some studies from the Brompton hospital, where PAF has been administered either in the skin or in guinea-pigs by the airways, have shown a very rapid decrease in both the neutrophil and eosinophil count after about 5 min. We have also observed this decreased leukocyte count following inhalation of PAF in subjects, however within 15 min the leukocyte count has returned to the base line and in fact may go above base line. It is not clear whether the mechanism for this is due to margination of these cells, possibly aggregation and rapid de-aggregation of the cells, but it's somewhat reminiscent of chemotactic deactivation.

Once the eosinophil has seen a chemotactic agent such as PAF, it will no longer be chemotactic to it. Similarly, in the human studies, after inhalation of PAF, there is a very rapid tachyphylaxis to PAF, both in terms of the decrease in pulmonary function and in the change in the leukocyte count. In other words, after leukopenia and eosinopenia have been induced by one dose of PAF then subsequent doses fail to induce further effects. I'd like to ask anybody here whether this rapid tachyphylaxis to PAF, both in the inhalation and on the leukocyte neutropenia and eosinopenia, could be due to a similar mechanism, as is seen in chemotaxis; namely: repeated use of the same chemotactic agent causing loss of effect.

Dahl: I think there is a great difference between the clinical situation and the situation where you inject zymosan or fMLP in the skin and have desensitization. In the human situation, where you rechallenge and rechallenge a site, you have the opposite effect. For example, the re-test situation, which has been known for 40 or 50 years. Injection of PPD in the skin causes a type 4 hypersensitivity reaction, with an early mononuclear infiltration followed by an eosinophilic infiltration. Injection of PPD for 3 or 4 days, causes a huge accumulation of eosinophils. In allergen-induced reactions, repeated allergen inhalation or injection causes eosinophil accumulation. So you wouldn't have desensitization. In studies on allergen challenge with Dr Venge we measured chemotactic factors in the blood and could predict from the variations in chemotactic activity if a late phase reaction would occur. If at several times during such a challenge the neutrophils and eosinophils are isolated from the blood and their response to chemotactic factors measured, the cells were deactivated. So chemotactic factors may activate certain cells which may be accumulated while other cells are deactivated. I don't know, I can't see any other explanation. But it's not always all cells that are deactivated and you are not, by repeating the allergen presentation to the body, deactivating all cells.

Colditz: Yes, I agree with your comments. In my experience the only stimulus that has been able repeatedly to cause accumulation of neutrophils in inflammatory lesions has been an immunologically driven inflammatory response, not one induced *in vivo* by a purified chemotactic factor. One other comment—the phenomenon that we have seen is not due to intravenous desensitization of the neutrophils. It is due to a site-specific desensitization to the chemotactic factors.

Dahl: Could I ask a question of Dr Townley? PAF may stimulate an eosinophil to produce LTC_4, and you say it activates the eosinophil. Have you looked to see if exposure of eosinophils to PAF induces PAF production from the eosinophil?

Townley: No, we haven't done that, although I think there is some evidence from the literature that PAF may induce PAF production.

Kay: Bob, can I ask you about your scheme that you showed at the end because, if I understand you correctly on the basis of your PMA experiments, you are suggesting that protein kinase C and the calcium pool somehow synergize for LTC_4 release. In fact, in the data you showed, you are going from about 5 ng up to about 6.6 ng, even with a hundred ng per ml PMA. So, I wondered first why you actually call that synergism. Another possible explanation could be a negative feedback of protein kinase C on phospholipase

C, which is known to exist in other systems, somehow altering the substrate availability for leukotriene. In other words, you're stopping arachidonic acid being diverted down non-5-lipoxygenase pathways.

Townley: Yes, that is an alternative possibility. The lowest concentration of PMA was actually more effective than the higher one. So, the response certainly wasn't dose related. Unfortunately, we didn't use lower concentrations of PMA to see if we could see a dose response.

Kay: What do you think the second messenger systems are with the more physiological triggers; for instance, IgG, IgE and complement with opsonized zymosan?

Townley: Well, I think the ultimate messenger is probably calcium, induced by inositol triphosphate or Ca^{++} combined with protein kinase C in direct stimulation. However, these avenues need to be further investigated.

Makino: In this discussion, we have received a great deal of information about chemotactic activity of PAF and the ability of PAF to attract eosinophils to the site of the inflammation. When we gave the PAF intrabronchially, we obtained maximal eosinophilic infiltration 6 h after PAF application, PAF is very easily metabolized, so, at the first contact with the cell membrane, PAF penetrates the membrane and probably PAF stimulates some cells to secrete something which attract the eosinophils. We find maximal eosinophilic infiltration 6 h after PAF application, 6 h after antigen challenge and also 6 h after fMLP inhalation in rabbits. So 6 h is a very critical time, but we don't know why.

Sanjar: I would like to direct a comment towards Dr Vadas. The last slide you showed was very interesting because we have some observations in animals which are quite similar. In lesions where there are eosinophils we rarely ever find neutrophils, and in lesions where there are neutrophils we rarely ever find eosinophils. If you see both cell types, it's at a transition time when neutrophils are decreasing and eosinophils are increasing. I wonder if rather than one cell inhibiting the other cell type, part of the explanation is actually that the stimulus prevents other cell types coming into the lesions. I would like to hear your comments on that.

Vadas: I have to think about it a bit. Well, it's quite complicated the mechanism of all this. The mechanism is partly an alteration in the affinity of the receptor for the chemoattractant. Following incubation, the cells lose the high affinity component of their fmet-leu-phe receptor. I think that's part of it. Now, I'm just trying to think of immobilizing cells in a lesion, how that could influence the influx of other cells. I don't know. What's your hypothesis?

Sanjar: As an animal pharmacologist, I am mostly interested in observations of what mediators do and it is a very constant observation that we never see the two cell types at the same time together. It is a fact which needs to be incorporated into any hypothesis and that's why I wanted to find out what your comments would be.

Vadas: I'll think about it over a few drinks tonight.

Wasserman: A series of studies done by David Bass many years ago looked at the ability of an *E. coli* abscess to inhibit eosinophilopoiesis and to decrease the eosinophil counts in parasitized animals. The studies also demonstrated that in the central part of a neutrophilic abscess, there were no eosinophils but at the periphery there were plenty of eosinophils. It may have to do with concentration gradients. These experiments used adrenalectomized animals, so, David Bass's view was that the absences of eosinophils in the abscess was not a glucocorticoid response but that there was a product, either of the bacterium or the neutrophil which inhibited the eosinophil. He didn't identify the inhibitor.

Gleich: We now have systems which will allow us to look at both eosinophil degranulation and neutrophil degranulation utilizing neutrophil elastase as a marker in studying typical allergic inflammation. Takoda Fujisawa has shown very clearly, just what was said a moment ago, that the eosinophil and neutrophil do not seem to keep company at all. There are very few neutrophils, you would see one or two neutrophils to 100 eosinophils in lesions of chronic allergic inflammation involving the upper airway. In the lower airway it's more complicated and possible infections in these lesions make interpretation more difficult.

Makino: I would like now to close this discussion. Thank you, Professor Townley.

7

Eosinophil Heterogeneity

T. Fukuda and S. Makino

Department of Allergy and Clinical Immunology,
Dokkyo University School of Medicine,
Tochigi 321-02, Japan

7.1 INTRODUCTION

Since the development of techniques to purify eosinophils by centrifugation on metrizamide or Percoll gradients (1, 2), a population of eosinophils of lower than normal density has been found and referred to as light-density or hypodense eosinophils. Hypodense eosinophils are present in the blood of patients with such eosinophilia-associated diseases as the hypereosinophilic syndrome, parasitism, allergy and neoplasia. Furthermore, it has been shown by many investigative groups that the hypodense eosinophils are functionally and morphologically distinct from the normodense eosinophils. During experiments using eosinophils purified on metrizamide or Percoll gradients, we also noticed that some of the eosinophils from patients with eosinophilia sedimented at densities lower than those of normal subjects. These observations prompted us to investigate the density distribution of eosinophils in health

Eosinophils in Asthma
ISBN 0-12-506452-7

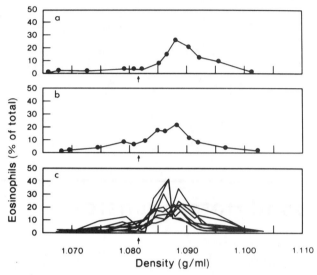

Fig. 1   Density distribution of eosinophils. (**a, b**) Profiles from 2 normal subjects; (**c**) profiles from 8 additional normal subjects. Results are shown as percentage of the total eosinophils recovered from the gradients. Each point represents 1 fraction. The arrows indicate 1.082 g/ml.

and disease in more detail, and the ultrastructural morphology of hypodense eosinophils. The results of those studies led to further experiments to attempt *in vitro* induction of hypodense eosinophils.

7.2   HETEROGENEITY OF EOSINOPHIL DENSITY

Eosinophils have the greatest density of human peripheral blood leukocytes. Figure 1 shows density distribution profiles of eosinophils obtained from ten normal individuals. Peak eosinophil densities were between 1.085 and 1.090 g/ml, with a mean of 1.0880 ± 0.0011 g/ml ($\bar{X}$ ± 1 SD). The density distribution profiles of 7 of the 10 normal subjects had inflection points near 1.082 g/ml, below which few eosinophils were found (Fig. 1a). In the remaining three normal subjects, although density distribution profiles had nadirs near 1.082 g/ml, a small population of eosinophils was found below 1.082 g/ml (Fig. 1b). On the basis of these findings, we defined hypodense eosinophils as cells lighter than 1.082 g/ml. The percentage of hypodense eosinophils in the normal subjects ranged from 1.2 to 22.8% with mean of 10.3%. Repeated determination of normal eosinophils density distribution using blood from

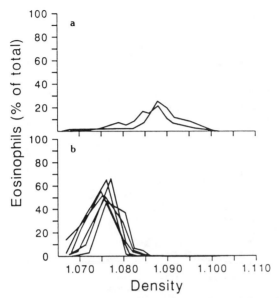

Fig. 2 Density distribution profiles of eosinophils. (**a**) Profiles from 2 representative normal subjects; (**b**) profiles from 6 patients with striking eosinophilia. Results are shown as percentage of the total eosinophils recovered from the gradients. Each point represents 1 fraction.

another healthy group also showed inflection points or nadirs near 1.082 g/ml, indicating that a density of 1.082 g/ml is a reproducible cut-off point. The investigators who used metrizamide gradients, referred to cells that sedimented in the lightest gradient fractions (in 18 to 23% metrizamide solutions) as hypodense eosinophils (3). This raised the question of whether or not cell populations separated according to these different definitions are the same. However, the percentage of hypodense eosinophils in normal subjects was approximately 10% by both methods, indicating that these two populations are probably the same.

Hypodense eosinophils are present in the blood of patients with eosinophilia-associated disease. Figure 2 shows the density distribution profiles of the eosinophils from six patients with striking eosinophilia. Four of these patients had hypereosinophilic syndrome (HES), one had episodic angiooedema and one had hepatitis. The peak density ranged from 1.075 to 1.078 g/ml, and the percentage of hypodense eosinophils was more than 90%. The density distribution profiles of eosinophils from the 10 patients with asthma could be divided into three groups as typified by the three profiles shown in Figure 3a–c; the remaining seven profiles are shown in Figure 3d.

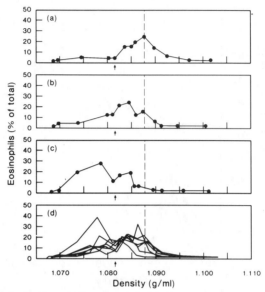

Fig. 3   Density distribution profiles of eosinophils from patients with asthma. (**a-c**) Profiles from 3 representative patients; (**d**) profiles from 7 additional patients. Results are shown as percentage of the total eosinophils recovered from the gradients. Each point represents 1 fraction. The arrows indicate 1.082 g/ml. The broken vertical lines indicate the mean peak density of eosinophils from the 10 normal subjects.

The mean of peak eosinophil density and the percentage of hypodense eosinophils in patients with asthma were 1.083 g/ml and 34.8%, respectively. The density profiles from patients with asthma seem to vary with time. In a representative case, the peak eosinophil density varied from 1.078 to 1.084 g/ml and the percentage of hypodense eosinophils varied from 49 to 30% during a period of 3 months. A positive correlation was usually observed between log-transformed peripheral blood eosinophil counts and the percentage of hypodense eosinophils (4). An exception to this rule was the blood eosinophils from the patients with chronic myelogenous leukaemia (CML) in remission stage. The density distribution analysis of the eosinophils from four patients with CML in remission revealed an increased number of hypodense eosinophils in the absence of blood eosinophilia.

Many hypodense eosinophils are present in the bronchoalveolar lavage fluids from asthmatics (5, 6). Bronchoalveolar lavage fluid and peripheral blood were obtained in parallel from five patients with asthma and their eosinophil density distributions were compared. As shown in Figure 4, in all cases bronchoalveolar eosinophils showed lower densities compared with those of

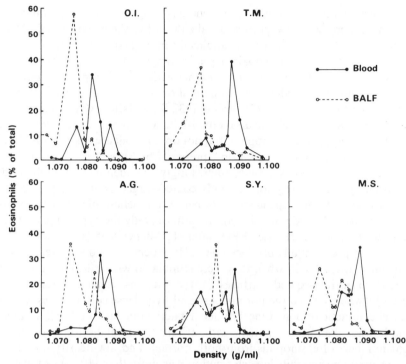

Fig. 4 Density distribution profiles of blood and bronchoalveolar eosinophils from 5 patients with asthma. Bronchoalveolar lavage fluid and peripheral blood were obtained in parallel and density distribution of the eosinophil was determined. Results are shown as percent of the total eosinophils recovered from the Percoll gradients. Each point represents 1 fraction.

blood eosinophils. Immature eosinophils in the bone marrow are also hypodense. Bone marrow cells were fractionated into 13 fractions according to density by using Percoll density gradients and differential counts of eosinophils according to the maturation stage were carried out in each fraction. Immature eosinophils with round nuclei were found only in the light-density fractions, while mature eosinophils were distributed over all fractions.

7.3 FUNCTIONAL HETEROGENEITY

A large number of functional differences between hypodense and normodense eosinophils has been reported. In other words, density heterogeneity seems to be associated with functional heterogeneity. A higher oxygen consumption (7) and an increased deoxyglucose uptake (8) in hypodense eosinophils have suggested that these cells are metabolically more active than normodense eosinophils. However, the impaired respiratory burst activity of hypodense eosinophils may reflect a previous *in vivo* activation (3). Compared to normodense eosinophils, hypodense eosinophils showed an increased expression of membrane receptors for Fcγ (7) and Fcε (23). Recent studies by Capron *et al.* (9) showed that a monoclonal antibody, BB10, was able to react with the Fcε receptor on hypodense eosinophils, but not on normodense eosinophils. Similarly, a monoclonal antibody, Eon7, prepared by Spry *et al.* (10) seems to react with hypodense eosinophils. Interestingly, hypodense eosinophils show enhanced cytoxic activity for antibody-coated targets. For example, it has been found that IgE-dependent cytotoxicity for helminthic larvae are restricted to these hypodense cells (8). In addition, only the hypodense eosinophils were able to release EPO after IgE-dependent activation (11). Eosinophils preferentially produce LTC_4. Hypodense eosinophils were found to produce more LTC_4 when they were stimulated with calcium ionophore A23187 (12), IgG-coated particles (13) or serum-treated zymosan (14). Recently, we compared the normodense and hypodense cells with respect to their chemotactic responsiveness to platelet activating factor (PAF). A blood sample was taken from a patient with striking eosinophilia to obtain sufficient numbers of eosinophils from both normal- and low-density fractions. The purity of eosinophils in each fraction was more than 90%. As shown in Figure 5, the hypodense cells showed a significantly greater chemotactic response to 30 nM PAF than did the normodense cells. Similar results were obtained from a subsequent experiment using highly purified hypodense and normodense eosinophils from another patient with marked eosinophilia. Thus, hypodense eosinophils may be activated cells and may represent the end result of the effects of the activating agents. Furthermore, the existence of hypodense eosinophils may partly explain the prior observation that there are metabolic differences among eosinophils from patients with hypereosinophilia of diverse causes (15).

7.4   ULTRASTRUCTURAL MORPHOLOGY OF HYPODENSE EOSINOPHILS

In spite of the increasing evidence of functional differences between the two subsets of eosinophils, there have been few data concerning the difference in ultrastructural morphology. We therefore investigated the ultrastructural

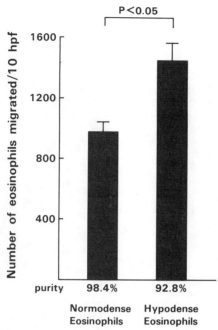

Fig. 5 Comparison of chemotactic response to platelet activating factor (30 nM) between normodense and hypodense eosinophils. Eosinophils used in this experiment were obtained from a patient with striking blood eosinophilia. Normodense and hypodense eosinophils were recovered from the fraction of a percoll gradient with densities of 1.0916 and 1.0797 g/ml, respectively. Values are the mean ± SE of single experiment in triplicate.

morphology of hypodense eosinophils to determine the morphologic basis of this low density. For this purpose, two sources of hypodense eosinophils were utilized: peripheral blood eosinophils from patients with HES and bronchoalveolar lavage fluid eosinophils from patients with asthma. As described above, more than 90% of the eosinophils from the peripheral blood of patients with HES are hypodense, while about 90% of the eosinophils from the peripheral blood of normal subjects are normodense. Such homogeneity of hypodense or normodense eosinophils allows observation of their ultrastructure without having to fractionate the cells. Figure 6b shows an electron-photomicrograph of a hypodense eosinophil obtained from a patient with HES. Although a similar number of granules are contained, the individual granules are obviously smaller than those of normal eosinophils (Fig. 6a). In addition to this finding, the eosinophils obtained from another patient consistently showed an increased number of lipid bodies as compared with normal subject eosinophils. To quantitate these findings, the number of granules per

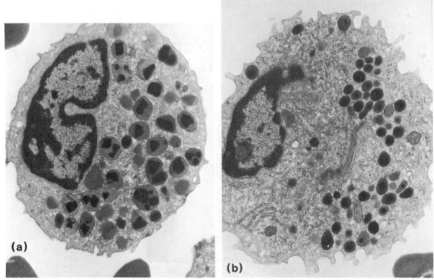

Fig. 6 Comparison of the morphology of normodense and hypodense eosinophils. (a) Normodense and (b) hypodense eosinophils contain similar numbers of granules, but the individual granules are smaller in the cells from the HES patients (× 17 500).

cell, and the cross-sectional areas of the eosinophils and their individual granules were determined. The analyses were based on a total of 174 eosinophils from three patients with HES and two normal individuals, using a computer program for digitizing areas. The total cellular area and the number of granules per cell were not significantly different for hypodense as compared with normodense eosinophils. However, the total granule area per cell and the percentage of cytoplasm occupied by granules were significantly lower in the hypodense eosinophil group. In this study (16), the major basic protein content per one million eosinophils was also determined. In agreement with the morphologic findings, the major basic protein content of hypodense eosinophils was significantly lower than that of normodense cells from normal subjects. Furthermore, the major basic protein content increases as cell density increases, suggesting that decrease in granule protein content may be one of the factors causing cell hypodensity.

In the next series of experiments we studied the ultrastructural morphology of hypodense eosinophils from the bronchoalveolar lavage fluids of patients with asthma, and compared it with that of blood eosinophils obtained from the same patients (6). In spite of the existence of a substantial percentage of hypodense eosinophils in asthmatic's peripheral blood, most of blood eosino-

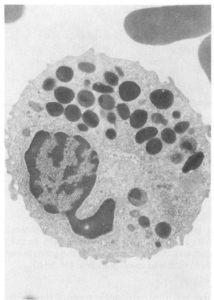

Fig. 7 Morphology of a blood eosinophil obtained from a patient with moderate asthma. The ultrastructure is essentially normal (× 7200).

phils showed almost normal ultrastructure (Fig. 7). On the other hand, bronchoalveolar eosinophils simultaneously obtained from the same patient consistently showed partial or complete lucency of the granule matrix (Fig. 8). These findings may explain the low density of bronchoalveolar eosinophils.

Thus, present studies clearly indicated that the ultrastructural morphology may differ depending on the type of underlying disease, or the stage of activation.

7.5 *IN VITRO* INDUCTION OF HYPODENSE EOSINOPHILS

As described above, the density distribution of peripheral blood eosinophils from patients with asthma varied with time. Moreover, there is a report that the proportion of hypodense eosinophils increased after antigen challenge in patients with asthma (17). These findings suggest a possibility that the mediators released into the bloodstream associated with immunological reaction may be responsible for the appearance of hypodense eosinophils. Indeed, in

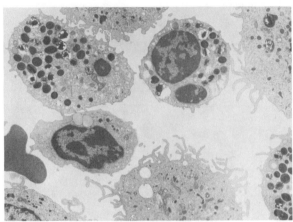

Fig. 8 Morphology of bronchoalveolar eosinophils simultaneously obtained from the same patient (Fig. 7). There are two eosinophils in this field. In the eosinophil on the right most granules display a partial or complete lucency of the granule matrix. The eosinophils on the left shows lucency of the matrix in some granules. (× 3840).

neutrophils, incubation with chemotactic agents has been shown to result in changes in cell density (18). For these reasons, we tested whether the *in vitro* interaction of human eosinophils with chemotactic agents may result in a change in density.

Leukocytes were obtained from a normal individual or a patient with eosinophilia. Half of these leukocytes were incubated with ECF-A tetrapeptide or platelet activating factor (PAF), while the remainder were incubated in the absence of a chemotactic agent and served as control cells. After 60 min of incubation at 37°C, cells were centrifuged on Percoll density gradients and the eosinophil density distribution was determined. Figure 9 shows the results of the experiments in which leukocytes were incubated with 30 nM of PAF for 60 min. The activation of eosinophils with PAF resulted in a marked reduction of cell density. Similar results were obtained in the experiment in which leukocytes were incubated with various concentrations of varyl-peptide. Stimulation of eosinophils with varyl-peptide resulted in a substantial shift of the cells towards a lower density relative to the unstimulated control cells. The effect of varyl-peptide was dose-dependent. To examine whether these changes in eosinophil density are due to degranulation of the cells or swelling of the cells, we performed the following experiments using purified human eosinophils. The eosinophils were incubated with PAF or varyl-peptide. After 60 min, the release of eosinophil granule protein into the supernatant and volume distribution of the eosinophils were determined. The release of eosinophil granule protein was determined by measurement of the

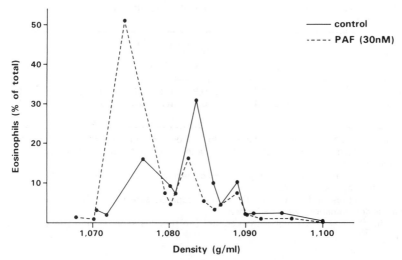

Fig. 9 Change in the density distribution of eosinophils following exposure to platelet activating factor. Leukocytes were incubated with platelet activating factor, at a concentration of 30 nM, for 30 min, centrifuged on Percoll density gradients, and the eosinophil density distribution was determined.

amount of eosinophil-derived neurotoxin (EDN) in the supernatant by the method described previously (19). Volume distribution of eosinophils was determined using a Coulter counter equipped with a volume analyser system by the method of O'Flaherty (20). Table 1 shows the effect of PAF at concentration of 1 μM to 1 nM on the release of EDN from human eosinophils. The incubation of eosinophils with PAF did not cause a significant release of EDN as compared to the control. Similar results were obtained when eosinophils were incubated with varyl-peptide. Figure 10 shows the change in volume distribution of eosinophils following exposure to PAF at a concentration of 30 nM. The incubation of eosinophils with PAF caused an increase in cell volume, suggesting the swelling of the cells. The incubation of eosinophils with varyl-peptide also caused an increase in eosinophil volume. Thus, the *in vitro* interaction of eosinophils with chemotactic agents caused changes in cell density and cell volume, but not degranulation.

Because the cell density is determined by the ratio of cell weight to cell volume, our findings of increase in cell volume not associated with the release of cellular components might explain the shift in eosinophil density towards lower values after exposure to chemotactic agents. In other words, changes in cell density and cell volume may be different measures of the same cellular response resulting from interaction with chemotactic factor. In addition, this

Table 1   Release of EDN from human eosinophils exposed to varying concentrations of PAF or LTB₄[a]

Stimulus	Concentration (M)				
	0	1×10^{-6}	1×10^{-7}	1×10^{-8}	1×10^{-9}
PAF	1.6 ± 0.4[b,c]	2.0 ± 0.3	1.8 ± 0.2	1.7 ± 0.3	1.6 ± 0.4
LTB₄	1.6 ± 0.4	1.5 ± 0.3	1.7 ± 0.4	1.7 ± 0.4	1.6 ± 0.2
A23187 1 µg/ml	13.0 ± 2.1[d]				

[a] Eosinophils (5 × 10⁵) were incubated with PAF or LTB₄ at the concentrations indicated, or with 1 µg/ml of A23187 for 60 min at 37°C, after which EDN release into the supernatant was determined.
[b] Results are expressed as percentage of total cellular content. Total cellular EDN content in 5 × 10⁵ eosinophils was 2379 ± 324 ng.
[c] All values represent the mean ± SEM of three separate experiments. In each experiment, duplicate determinations were performed.
[d] Significantly ($p < 0.05$) higher than control (no stimulus added) using t-test for paired data.

mechanism, together with an increase in lipid bodies, might explain the lower density of peripheral blood eosinophils from patients with asthma. As described above, although most of blood eosinophils showed almost normal ultrastructure, a considerable number of hypodense eosinophils were present in the peripheral blood of the patients with asthma.

Eosinophilopoietin also seems to be involved in the appearance of the hypodense eosinophils. Recently, it has been shown that granulocyte-macrophage colony stimulating factor (GM-CSF), which is known to induce

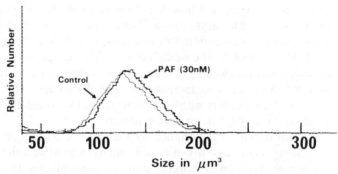

Fig. 10   Volume distribution curve of eosinophils incubated with platelet activating factor. Purified human eosinophils were incubated with or without platelet activating factor, at a concentration of 30 nM, at 37°C for 60 min, and volume distribution of the eosinophils was determined using a Coulter counter equipped with a volume analyser system.

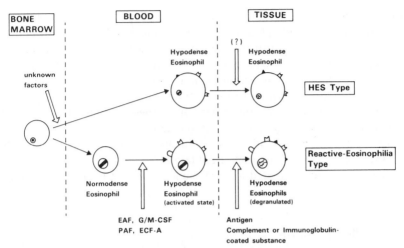

Fig. 11   The hypodense eosinophil hypothesis (see text for explanation).

granulocytosis with eosinophilia, regulates human eosinophil viability, density and function (21). Normodense human eosinophils cultured with recombinant human GM-CSF in the presence of mouse 3T3 fibroblasts became hypodense and had an augmented capacity to generate LTC_4 and to kill *S. mansoni* larvae.

7.6   HYPODENSE EOSINOPHIL HYPOTHESIS

It is still unclear whether the hypodense eosinophils are derived from a separate population of bone marrow precursor cells or are activated by the disease process. However, the latter is more likely, because activation of normodense eosinophils by various substances, such as chemotactic factors, eosinophil-activating factor (EAF) (22) and GM-CSF, can result in many of the features of hypodense eosinophils.

Figure 11 shows our hypothesis concerning the appearance of hypodense eosinophils. According to this hypothesis, there exist at least two types of hypodense eosinophils. One is the HES-type hypodense eosinophil which is characterized by smaller granules. The other is the reactive eosinophilia-type hypodense eosinophil characterized by the presence of the findings of degranulation. Smaller granules and lower MBP content in HES-type hypodense eosinophils may be due to abnormal maturation in bone marrow. Unknown factors produced related to the disease process may be responsible for this possible abnormal maturation. Reactive-type hypodense eosinophils may represent the end result of the effect of the various agents. When normodense eosinophils are exposed to various mediators released into the bloodstream associated with the disease process, they become hypodense probably due to cell swelling or increased formation of lipid bodies. These hypodense eosinophils show an increased number of cell surface receptors, enhanced cytotoxicity and increased chemotactic activity. After these eosinophils arrive at the inflammatory sites, they may be further activated probably by the local factors such as antigen, and/or complement or antibody-coated substance, and then may finally release their granule components.

Further research is needed for better understanding of eosinophil heterogeneity.

Acknowledgements

A part of this research was performed under the direction of Prof. Gerald J. Gleich of the Mayo Clinic. The electronphotomicrographs in Figure 6a, b were through courtesy of Dr Margot S. Peters of the Mayo Clinic. We thank the organizers of the symposium for inviting us to participate and for their kind and most generous hospitality.

REFERENCES

1. Vadas, M. A., David, J. R., Butterworth, A., Pisani, N. T. and Siongok, T. A. (1979). A new method for the purification of human eosinophils and neutrophils, and a comparison of the ability of these cells to damage schistosomula of *Schistosoma mansoni*. *J. Immunol.* **122**, 1228–1236.
2. Gartner, I. (1980). Separation of human eosinophils in density gradients of polyvinylpyrrolidone-coated silica gel (Percoll). *Immunology* **40**, 133–136.
3. Prin, L., Charon, J., Capron, M., Gosset, P., Taelman, H., Tonnel, A. B. and Capron, A. (1984). Heterogeneity of human eosinophils. II. Variability of respiratory burst activity related to cell density. *Clin. Exp. Immunol.* **57**, 735–742.
4. Fukuda, T., Dunnette, S. L., Reed, C. E., Ackerman, S. J., Peters, M. S. and Gleich, G. J. (1985). Increased numbers of hypodense eosinophils in the blood of patients with bronchial asthma. *Am. Rev. Respir. Dis.* **132**, 981–985.
5. Prin, L., Capron, M., Gosset, P., Wallaert, B., Kusnierz, J. P., Bletry, O., Tonnel, A. B. and Capron, A. (1986). Eosinophilic lung disease: immunological studies of blood and alveolar eosinophils. *Clin. Exp. Immunol.* **63**, 249–257.
6. Fukuda, T., Numao, T., Akutsu, I. and Makino, S. (1987). Comparison of density distribution and ultrastructural morphology of blood and bronchoalveolar eosinophils in patients with asthma. *The Cell* (in Japanese) **19**, 192–198.

7. Winqvist, I., Olofsson, T., Olsson, I., Persson, A. and Hallberg, T. (1982). Altered density, metabolism and surface receptors of eosinophils in eosinophilia. *Immunology* **47**, 531–539.

8. Prin, L., Capron, M., Tonnel, A. B., Bletry, O. and Capron, A. (1983). Heterogeneity of human peripheral blood eosinophils: variability in cell density and cytotoxic ability in relation to the level and the origin of hypereosinophilia. *Int. Archs. Allergy appl. Immun.* **72**, 336–346.

9. Capron, M., Jouault, T., Prin, L., Joseph, M., Ameisen, J. C., Butterworth, A. E., Parin, J. P., Kusnierz, J. P. and Capron, A. (1986). Functional study of a monoclonal antibody to IgE Fc receptors (FcεR2) of eosinophils, platelets, and macrophages. *J. Exp. Med.* **164**, 72–89.

10. Tai, P.-C., Bakes, D. M., Barkans, J. R. and Spry, C. J. F. (1985). Plasma membrane antigens on light density and activated human blood eosinophils. *Clin. Exp. Immunol.* **60**, 427–436.

11. Khalife, J., Capron, M., Cesbron, J. Y., Tai, P.-C., Taelman, H., Prin, L. and Capron, A. (1986). Role of specific IgE antibodies in peroxidase (EPO) release from human eosinophils. *J. Immunol.* **137**, 1659–1664.

12. Kajita, T., Yui, Y., Mita, H., Taniguchi, N., Saito, H., Mishima, T., and Shida, T. (1985). Release of leukotriene C_4 from human eosinophils and its relation to the cell density. *Int. Archs. Allergy Appl. Immun.* **78**, 406–410.

13. Shaw, R. J., Walsh, G. M., Cromwell, O., Moqbel, R., Spry, C. J. F. and Kay, A. B. (1985). Activated human eosinophils generate SRS-A leukotrienes following IgG-dependent stimulation. *Nature* **316**, 150–152.

14. Kauffman, H. F., Belt, van der B., Monchy de J. G. R., Boelens, H., Koeter, G. H. and Vries, de K. (1987). Leukotriene C_4 production by normal-density and low-density eosinophils of atopic individuals and other patients with eosinophilia. *J. Allergy Clin. Immunol.* **79**, 611–619.

15. Pincus, S. H., Schooley, W. R., DiNapoli, A. M. and Broder, S. (1981). Metabolic heterogeneity of eosinophils from normal and hypereosinophilic patients. *Blood* **58**, 1175–1181.

16. Peters, M. S., Gleich, G. J., Dunnette, S. L. and Fukuda, T. (1989). Ultrastructural study of eosinophils from patients with the hypereosinophilic syndrome: a morphologic basis of hypodense eosinophils. *Blood* **71**, 780–785.

17. Frick, W. E., Sedgwick, J. B. and Busse, W. W. (1988). The appearance of hypodense eosinophils (HE) in late-phase asthma [abstract]. *J. All. Clin. Immunol.* **81**, 208.

18. Pember, S. O., Barnes, K. C., Brandt, S. J. and Kinkade, J. M. (1983). Density heterogeneity of neutrophilic polymorphonuclear leukocytes: gradient fractionation and relationship to chemotactic stimulation. *Blood* **61**, 1105–1115.

19. Fukuda, T., Ackerman, S. J., Reed, C. E., Peters, M. S., Dunnette, S. L. and Gleich, G. J. (1985). Calcium ionophore A23187 causes calcium-dependent cytolytic degranulation in human eosinophils. *J. Immunol.* **135**, 1349–1356.

20. O'Flaherty, J. T., Kreutzer, D. L. and Ward, P. A. (1977). Neutrophil aggregation and swelling induced by chemotactic agents. *J. Immunol.* **119**, 232–239.

21. Owen, W. F., Rothenberg, M. E., Silberstein, D. S., Gasson, J. C., Stevens, R. L., Austen, K. F. and Soberman, R. J. (1987). Regulation of human eosinophil viability, density, and function by granulocyte/macrophage colony-stimulating factor in the presence of 3T3 fibroblasts. *J. Exp. Med.* **166**, 129–141.

22. Fitzharris, P., Moqbel, R., Thorne, K. J. I., Richardson, B. A., Hartnell, A., Crom-

well, O., Butterworth, A. E. and Kay, A. B. (1986). The effects of eosinophil activating factor on IgG-dependent sulphidopeptide leukotriene generation by human eosinophils. *Clin. Exp. Immunol.* **66**, 673–680.
23. Capron, M., Spiegelberg, H. L., Prin, L., Bennich, H., Butterworth, A. E., Pierce, R. J., Aliouaissi, M. and Capron, A. (1984). Role of IgE receptors in effector function of human eosinophils. *J. Immunol.* **132**, 462–468.

8

Changes in the Number of Hypodense Eosinophils and the Expression of Complement Receptors of Eosinophils by Allergen Inhalation and Steroid Therapy in Patients with Bronchial Asthma

M. Suko, H. Okudaira, T. Miyamoto and T. Shida*

Department of Medicine and Physical Therapy, Faculty of Medicine, University of Tokyo, Japan

*Sagamihara National Hospital Center for Rheumatology and Allergy, Japan

---

8.1 INTRODUCTION

Allergen inhalation developed an immediate asthmatic reaction in atopic patients with bronchial asthma, accompanied by increases in the numbers of hypodense eosinophils and in the expression of complement receptors of

Eosinophils in Asthma
ISBN 0-12-506452-7

normodense eosinophils in peripheral blood. Chemical mediators such as ECF-A, histamine and PAF increased both the number of hypodense eosinophils and the expression of complement receptors after the incubation of normodense eosinophils *in vitro*.

Corticosteroid therapy was seen to reduce the number of hypodense eosinophils and the expression of complement receptors of eosinophils in patients with asthmatic attacks. These observations suggested that activation of eosinophils during allergen-induced immediate asthmatic response might be important for the induction of late asthmatic reactions.

Attention has been paid to the role of eosinophils in the pathogenesis of bronchial asthma. Recent studies have shown increased numbers of eosinophils in the blood and in the bronchoalveolar lavage in patients with allergen-induced late phase asthmatic reaction (1, 2). It is well known that there is a heterogeneity in eosinophil with respect to its structure and its function. Recently Fukuda and Gleich reported that asthmatic patients have increased numbers of hypodense eosinophils compared with normal subjects (3). We therefore studied eosinophil heterogeneity in relation to allergen-induced asthmatic response and corticosteroid therapy.

8.2   MATERIAL AND METHODS

Circulating eosinophils were separated from heparinized blood by the combination of dextran sedimentation and metrizamide density gradients, according to the methods described by Prin *et al.* (4).

After the separation, numbers of eosinophils were counted in each cell fraction with different density (Fig. 1) and the expression of complement receptors of eosinophils were measured by counting rosettes formed with sheep red cell sensitized with IgM and coated with fresh human serum, abbreviated EAC rosettes.

8.3   RESULTS

8.3.1   Density distribution profiles of eosinophils

The density distribution of eosinophils from an asthmatic subject became smaller compared with that from a healthy subject. This is consistent with the findings of Fukuda *et al.* that the number of hypodense eosinophils increased

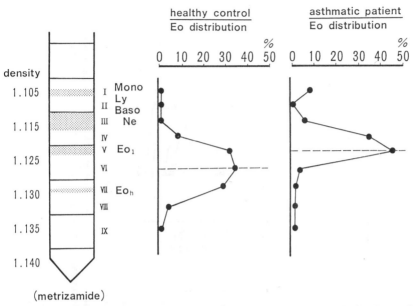

Fig. 1 Leukocytes were sedimented with dextran and laid on metrizamide density gradients. Eosinophils in each fraction with different density were counted for the calculation of density distribution. Mono: monocyte; Ly: lymphocyte; Baso: basophil; Ne: neutrophil; Eo_l: eosinophil with low density; Eo_h: eosinophils with high density.

in asthmatic patients (4). In the present study, we refer to eosinophils obtained from metrizamide gradients with 18–20% solution as hypodense eosinophils and those from 23 to 24% metrizamide solutions as normodense eosinophils.

8.3.2   Changes in the Numbers of Hypodense Eosinophils and the Expression of Complement Receptors of Eosinophils during Allergen-induced Immediate Asthmatic Reactions

Eleven asthmatic patients who were sensitive to house dust mites were made to inhale house dust in stepwise increasing concentrations until a minimum fall of 20% was reached in forced expiratory volume in one second (Fig. 2).

Venous blood was withdrawn before and 60 min after allergen inhalation and examined for hypodense eosinophils and complement receptors of eosinophils.

Allergen inhalation did not show any change in the percentage of eosinophils in leukocytes in blood. However, the hypodense eosinophils signifi-

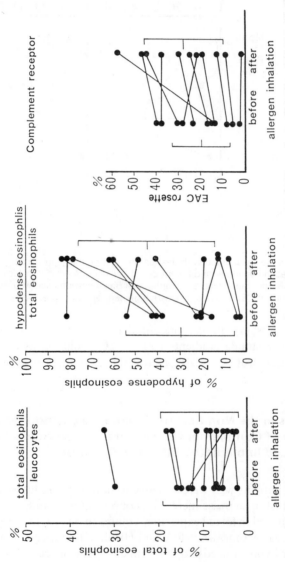

Fig. 2 House dust mite-sensitive asthmatic subjects were made inhale house dust until a minimum fall of 20% in forced expiratory volume in one second. Before and after the inhalation, percentages of whole and hypodense eosinophils and the expression of complement receptors were evaluated.

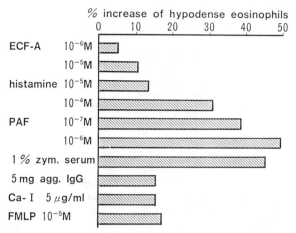

Fig. 3 Eosinophils with normodensity were incubated for 30 min at 37°C without or with various doses of ECF-A, histamine, PAF (platelet activating factor), 1% zym serum, Ca I (calcium ionophore) or FMLP. After the incubation, eosinophils were laid again on density gradient and centrifuged. After the centrifugation, changes in the percentage of hypodense eosinophils were examined.

cantly increased in number and the expression of complement receptors of eosinophils had a tendency to be enhanced after allergen inhalation.

8.3.3 *In vitro* Effect of Chemical Mediators on the Density Distribution of Eosinphils and the Expression of Complement Receptors of Eosinophils

Normodense eosinophils were incubated at 37°C for up to 30 min with ECF-A, histamine or PAF (Fig. 3). After the incubation, eosinophils were washed once and laid over the metrizamide density gradients again, followed by centrifugation for 45 min.

There was a time-dependent increase in the number of hypodense eosinophils after the incubation with PAF of 10^{-7} M concentration. Hypodense eosinophils appeared after only 2 min incubation and their numbers increased gradually. After 15 min incubation, most of the normodense eosinophils became hypodense.

Dose-dependent increases were also observed in the number of hypodense eosinophils after the incubation with ECF-A (10^{-6} M, 10^{-5} M), histamine (10^{-5} M, 10^{-4} M) or PAF (10^{-7} M, 10^{-6} M) (Fig. 3). PAF was the most potent substance to yield hypodense eosinophils from normodense eosinophils.

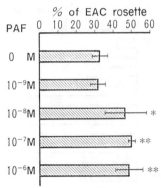

Fig. 4 Eosinophils with normodensity were incubated with PAF at different doses for 30 min at 37°C. After the incubation, EAC rosettes formation of eosinophils were examined (* $p < 0.05$; ** $p < 0.01$).

Complement receptors of eosinophils were enhanced by PAF treatment *in vitro*. More than 10^{-8} M of PAF significantly increased the percentage of EAC rosettes formation of eosinophils (Fig. 4).

8.3.4   Effect of Corticosteroid Therapy on the Absolute Number of Circulating Eosinophils and the Expression of Complement Receptors of Eosinophils.

We started corticosteroid therapy with eight patients with severe asthmatic attack, using dripped infusions of 100 mg hydrocortisone every day for 7 days (Fig. 5). Absolute numbers of circulating eosinophils, hypodense eosinophils and the expression of complement receptor were estimated before and after the corticosteroid therapy.

On the seventh day, when the asthmatic state of all patients was markedly improved, there were reductions in absolute numbers of eosinophils, hypodense eosinophils and the expression of complement receptors of eosinophils (Fig. 5).

8.4   DISCUSSION

In the present study we have shown that allergen inhalation induced increases in the number of hypodense eosinophils and in the expression of com-

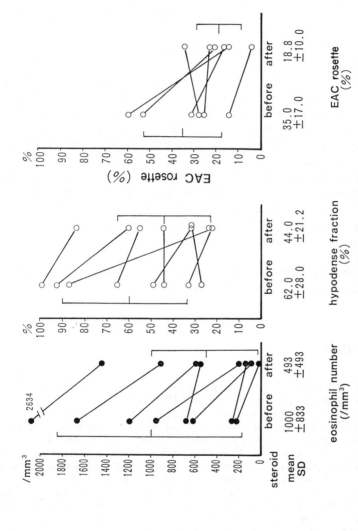

Fig. 5 Patients in asthmatic attack were treated with hydrocortisone every day for 7 days. Peripheral eosinophils were studied before and after the treatment for evaluating absolute numbers of whole eosinophils, percentages of hypodense eosinophils and the expression of complement receptors.

plement receptors of eosinophils in patients with bronchial asthma. These observations are consistent with the finding of Kay and his co-workers that there was an increase in the expression of circulating neutrophil and monocyte complement receptors after allergen induced asthma (5).

They also demonstrated that chemoattractants enhanced the expression of neutrophil and monocyte complement *in vitro* (6). Based on these observations, they propose that these inflammatory cells are activated by inflammatory mediators derived from mast cells in the bronchi.

We have also demonstrated mast cell associated mediators such as ECF-A, histamine and PAF increased the number of hypodense eosinophils and the expression of complement receptors of eosinophils *in vitro* and it is therefore possible that circulating eosinophils are activated to become hypodense and to have more complement receptors *in vivo*, by such mediators released from mast cells during allergen-induced immediate asthmatic reaction. These activated eosinophils might be more available for following stimuli and play a role in the allergen-induced late asthmatic reaction.

We have shown that corticosteroid therapy reduced not only the number of whole eosinophils but the number of hypodense eosinophils and the expression of complement receptors of eosinophils. This is consistent with an observation of Gin and Kay, who demonstrated that neutrophil and monocyte expression of complement receptors was decreased by corticosteroid therapy (7).

These findings may provide a new insight into the mechanisms of beneficial effect of corticosteroid therapy on bronchial asthma.

REFERENCES

1. Durham, S. R. and Kay, A. B. (1985). Eosinophils, bronchial hyperreactivity and late-phase asthmatic reactions. *Clin. Allergy* **15**, 411–418.
2. de Monchy, J. G. R., Kauffman, H. F., Venge, P., Koeter, G. H., Jansen, H. M., Sluiter, H. J. and de Vries, K. (1985). Bronchoalveolar eosinophilia during allergen-induced late asthmatic reactions. *Am. Rev. Respir. Dis.* **131**, 373–376.
3. Fukuda, T., Dunnette, S. L., Reed, C. E., Ackermand, S. J., Peters, M. S. and Gleich, G. L. (1985). Increased numbers of hypodense eosinophils in the blood of patients with bronchial asthma. *Am. Rev. Respir. Dis.* **132**, 981–985.
4. Prin, L., Charon, J., Capron, M., Gosset, P., Taelman, H., Tonnel, A. B. and Capron, A. (1984). Heterogeneity of human eosinophils. II. Variability of respiratory burst activity related to cell density. *Clin. Exp. Immunol.* **57**, 735–742.
5. Durham, S. R., Carroll, M., Walsh, G. M. and Kay, A. B. (1984). Leukocyte activation in allergen-induced late-phase asthmatic reactions. *New Engl. J. Med.* **29**, 1398–1402.

6. Kay, A. B., Glass, E. J. and Salter, D. G. (1979). Leucoattractants enhance complement receptors on human phagocytic cells. *Clin. Exp. Immunol.* **38**, 294–299.

7. Gin, W. and Kay, A. B. (1986). The effect of corticosteroids on monocyte and neutrophil activation in bronchial asthma. *J. Allergy Clin. Immunol.* **78**, 675–682.

9

Platelet Factor 4 has Chemotactic Activity for Eosinophils and Augments Fcγ and Fcε Receptor Expression on Eosinophils

J. Chihara and S. Nakajima

4th Department of Internal Medicine,
Kinki University School of Medicine,
Onohigashi Osakasayama, Osaka 589, Japan

9.1 INTRODUCTION

Platelets have been implicated as mediators of inflammatory and allergic reactions. Platelet activation has been associated with IgG and IgE antibody-related immune reactions (1) (2).

Platelet factor 4 (PF4) is stored in the α-granules of human platelets (3). Immunological stimuli such as immune complexes evoked the release of PF4 (1) (4) (5). Indeed, increases of PF4 in plasma in asthmatic attack and other allergic reactions were reported by some investigations (1) (4) (6) (7) (8). These findings suggest that PF4 may play a role in bronchial asthma as well

Eosinophils in Asthma
ISBN 0-12-506452-7

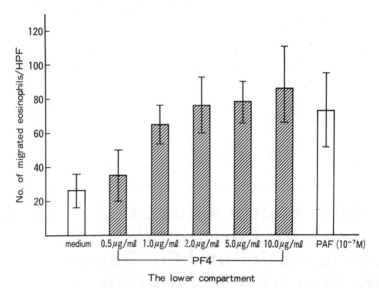

Fig. 1   PF4 has chemotactic activity for eosinophils. Eosinophil chemotaxis toward PF4 was observed at PF4 concentration of 1 μg/ml.

as eosinophils. Eosinophil–platelet interactions in allergic diseases, especially bronchial asthma is therefore a very important role in their pathogenesis. In this study, the effects of PF4 on eosinophils were investigated.

9.2   MATERIALS AND METHODS

9.2.1   Eosinophil Isolation

Leukocyte-rich plasma, obtained by dextran sedimentation of blood was applied to a discontinuous density gradient from 22 to 25% metrizamide in Tyrode's gel/DNase (9). Following centrifugation at $1000\,G$ for 30 min at 22°C, the eosinophil-rich fraction was retained, washed in Hank's balanced salt solution (HBSS) and resuspended in HBSS containing 10% FCS. The preparation of eosinophils usually revealed eosinophil purity of more than 91%.

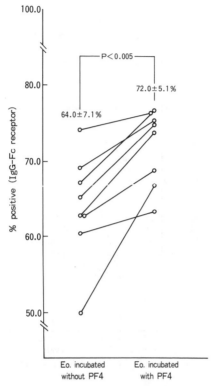

Fig. 2   The effect of incubation with PF4 (2.5 μg/ml) for 30 min at 37°C on IgG-Fc receptor of eosinophils.

9.2.2   Assay of Eosinophil Chemotactic Activity

Eosinophil chemotactic activity was assessed using a modified Boyden chamber method. The cell counts were adjusted 1×10^6/ml, and 0.2 ml was placed in the upper compartment of blind well chamber, 0.1 ml of various concentrations of PF4 (0.5 μg/ml, 1 μg/ml, 2 μg/ml, 5 μg/ml, 10 μg/ml) (Sigma Chemical Company, Lot No. 47F-9483) were placed in the lower compartment. After a 60 min incubation, the micropore filters (5 μm pore size) were removed, fixed, and stained by the May-Grünwald-Giemsa technique, and the number of eosinophils that had migrated through the filter was counted. The number of eosinophils in ten high power fields was counted. The samples were assayed in triplicate.

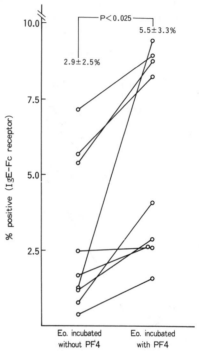

Fig. 3   The effect of incubation with PF4 (2.5 μg/ml) for 30 min at 37°C on IgE-Fc receptor of eosinophils.

9.2.3   Assay of IgG-Fc Receptor and IgE-Fc Receptor on Eosinophils

IgG-Fc receptor and IgE-Fc receptor on eosinophils were analysed by monoclonal antibodies. As monoclonal antibody anti-IgE-Fc receptor, H107(CD23) was used (10) (11). After indirect immunofluorescence labelling, eosinophils were assayed for their reactivity by flow cytometry (Orth-Spectrum III).

Results were expressed as both positive percentages of eosinophils and fluorescence intensity measured by fluorescence histogram.

9.3   RESULTS AND DISCUSSION

The chemotactic activity of PF4 for eosinophils and its relationship with PF4 concentrations are illustrated in Figure 1.

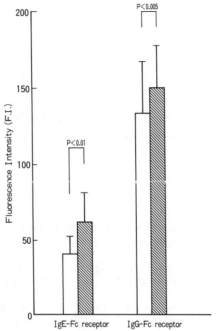

Fig. 4   Fluorescence intensity determined by flow cytometer (Ortho-Spectrum III) of eosinophils incubated with PF4 (hatched bars) and without PF4 (open bars).

Eosinophils chemotaxis toward lower compartments containing PF4 were observed at PF4 concentrations of 0.5 μg/ml in some cases but clearly observed at PF4 concentrations of 1.0 μg/ml. At more than 2.0 μg/ml, chemotactic response of eosinophils toward PF4 was nearly equal or more striking than that using platelet activating factor (PAF) at 10^{-7} M concentration, as a positive control, which is seemed to be most striking chemotactic factor for eosinophils *in vitro*.

On the other hand, IgG-Fc receptor expression on eosinophil was increased as expressed by percentages of positive eosinophils (Figure 2). IgE-Fc receptor expression on eosinophils was also increased (Figure 3).

Furthermore, fluorescence intensity of both IgG-Fc receptor and IgE-Fc receptor on eosinophils after incubation of PF4 were higher intensity than those without PF4 (Figure 4).

Our present results suggest that PF4 released from activated platelets may serve to attract eosinophils to the site of allergic reactions and augment eosinophil function via immunoglobulin. Thereby, interaction between eosinophils and platelets may play some important roles in the profile of bronchial asthma and other allergic reactions.

Acknowledgement

We wish to thank Dr J. Yodoi for providing the anti-FcεR$_2$ antibody (H107) and Miss Y. Hiraike for typing the manuscript.

REFERENCES

1. Knauer, K. A., Lichtenstein, L. M., Adkinsor, N. F. and Fish, J. E. (1981). Platelet activation during antigen-induced airway reactions in asthmatic subject. *N. Engl. J. Med.* **304**, 1404.
2. Halonen, M., and Pinckard, R. N. (1975). Intravascular effects of IgE antibody upon basophils, neutrophils, platelets, and blood coagulation in the rabbit. *J. Immunol.* **115**, 519.
3. Ryo, R., Proffitt, R. T. and Deuel, T. F. (1980). Human platelets factor 4: subcellular localization and characteristics of release from intact platelets. *Throm. Res.* **17**, 629.
4. Kaplan, K. L. and Owen, J. (1981). Plasma levels of β-thromboglobulin and platelet factor 4 as indices of platelet activation in vivo. *Blood* **57**, 199.
5. McManus, L. M., Morley, C. A., Levine, S. P. and Pinckard, R. N. (1979). Platelet activating factor (PAF) induces release of platelet factor 4 (PF4). *J. Immunol.* **123**, 2835.
6. Gresele, P., Todisco, T., Merante, F. and Nenci, G. G. (1982). Platelet activation and allergic asthma. *N. Engl. J. Med.* **306**, 549.
7. Metzger, W. J., Hunninghake, G. W. and Richerson, H. B. (1985). Late asthmatic responses: inquiry into mechanisms and significance. *Clin. Rev. Allergy* **3**, 145.
8. Johnson, C. E., Belfield, P. W., Davis, S., Cooke, N. J., Spencer, A. and Davies, J. A. (1986). Platelet activation during exercise induced asthma: effect of prophylaxis with cromoglycate and salbutamol. *Thorax* **41**, 290.
9. Vadas, M. A., David, J. R., Butterworth, A., Pisani, N. T. and Siongok, T. A. (1979). A new method for the purification of human eosinophils and neutrophils, and a comparison of the ability of those cells to damage schistosomula of schistosoma mansoni. *J. Immunol.* **122**, 1228.
10. Noro, N., Yashioka, A., Adachi, M., Yasuda, K., Masuda, T. and Yodoi, J. (1986). Monoclonal antibody (H107) inhibiting IgE binding to Fcε R($+$) human lymphocytes. *J. Immunol.* **137**, 1258.
11. Ikuta, K., Takami, M., Won Kim, C., Honjo, T., Miyoshi, T., Tagaya, Y., Kawabe, T. and Yodoi, J. (1987). Human lymphocyte Fc receptor for IgE: Sequence homology of its cloned cDNA with animal lectins. *Proc. Natl. Acad. Sci. USA.* **84**, 819.

DISCUSSION

Vargaftig (Chairman)

Gleich: Dr Fukuda's work would suggest that there are two mechanisms by which one might generate hypodense eosinophils. In the studies on patients with a hypereosinophilic syndrome, it could be due to premature release from the marrow. Alternatively, in your second schema, you identified several possibilities, such as swelling of the cells or perhaps a decrease in the cell density due to inclusion of light-density lipids within the cytoplasmic volume. Yet a third mechanism could be partial degranulation, and it seems to me that the results which Monique Capron presented yesterday would not be inconsistent with this possibility. Perhaps you'd like to comment Monique.

Capron: No, I totally agree with the different possibilities and I also think that there is not only one kind of hypodense eosinophil. When we look at different tissues such as kidneys or stomach, we have very different EM pictures. So I think that the mechanisms might be different in different tissues.

Gleich: So, you would agree that there are maybe many different kinds of heterogeneous eosinophils, or perhaps one might put it slightly differently, that the hypodense subset could be contributed to by manifold processes.

Wasserman: It actually may be a continuum because if you look at the lovely picture of the progressive changes from PAF, you can see that the density of the eosinophils changes increasingly with time. We won't get the slide back, but if you notice that the control in the 15 minutes without PAF are very stable, yet within 2 minutes not only is there a second band but even the dense band is somewhat less dense than the control band; and the distance between the two continues to increase throughout the incubation, suggesting that there may be a swelling initially and a degranulation subsequentially, and that these are maybe two processes being intermingled as that happens.

Gleich: I'd like to bring up a point which Dr Fukuda didn't dwell on but which none the less was clear from the electron photomicrograph of a bronchobiopsy in which you showed one eosinophil which was intact and an adjacent eosinophil which appeared to have undergone some destruction with release of membrane bound granules throughout the tissue. We have made the same observation repeatedly in skin biopsies and more recently in a pedigree of patients with an association between mental deficiency and eosinophilia with florid cutaneous lesions. We have seen enormous numbers of eosinophils which had degenerated and released membrane-bound granules within the tissues. Now, I was curious to know whether other persons have observed this, because we wonder whether or not, at least in some cases, certain stimuli may actually cause a toxic degeneration of the eosinophil. In other words, certain stimuli may actually cause death of an eosinophil. In the laboratory we refer to this as the kamikaze hypothesis.

Capron: I think I can answer this question. When we look at the levels of the parasite killing after one day for instance, consistently we see lysed eosinophils and degeneration at the contact of targets.

Vargaftig: We have similar pictures of degenerative eosinophils 24 h after PAF in guinea-pigs.

Vadas: May I comment on this. Actually, we spent some time making eosinophils and neutrophils targets to killing by themselves, and we found them to be very resistant, whereas you could kill them by other cells. So when you chromium label an eosinophil and ask another eosinophil to kill it, it can't. However, it can kill other cells and can be killed by T cells, for example. So, there seems to be a resistance for homologous damaging mechanisms. We didn't publish this, but it was reasonable data. I have a question. When you observe the hypodense eosinophils in hypereosinophilic syndrome, you could make a calculation by looking at the density of the granules and see if the decrease in the size of the granules allows you to calculate the change in density. Can you account for the change in density by the decreased volume of granules?

Fukuda: Yes, you mean the size of granules.

Vadas: Well, you say that hypodensity is due to small granules. I'm asking: does it mathematically add up?

Fukuda: What do you mean by mathematically adding up?

Vadas: Well, you know granule density and granule number so you can calculate the mass of granules per cell. You showed that the volume of the hypodense and the normodense cells is the same. It's just like a handbag, in one instance you have big coins, in the other instance you have small coins, so the handbag is lighter. I'm wondering whether in fact the lighter density is due to the coins or is it a paraphenomenon due to something else?

Gleich: It seems to be due to the size of the coins. One slide which Dr Fukuda showed indicated that there was a relationship between the quantity of MBP which one might take to be an indirect measure of the weight of the coins. As the quantity of MBP went up, the density went up. We would take that as consistent, although surely not proving that hypothesis.

Capron: I have a question for the two speakers. I was interested by the changes in the density of eosinophils in the same patient according to the time. But I have not noticed in which way the change occurred. Were the eosinophils hypodense first? Did this patient receive corticosteroid therapy?

Fukuda: The patient didn't take glucocorticoids.

Gleich: That's a very interesting one. Takeshi did comparable studies on normal individuals. Normal individuals stay the same; one subject didn't change much over about 8 months. The percentage of hypodense eosinophils stayed the same. In contrast, asthmatic patients appeared to vary. Now the hypothesis that one might entertain is that this variation would be in association with changes in the severity of the asthma. But that's a rather difficult study to do, and today, at least we haven't done it in our lab; maybe someone here has looked at this, to test the hypothesis that the spontaneous alterations in the severity of chronic asthma can be associated with the changes in the number of hypodense eosinophils. I think that would be a most intriguing hypothesis to test.

Suko: Yes, I think the distribution patterns are very changeable, depending on the asthmatic state.

de Monchy: We have not looked at several stages in the disease but we have looked before and after allergen challenge. Twenty-four hours after challenge, the number of eosinophils in this group of patients, who had both early and late reactions, increased dramatically. But the percentage of hypodense eosinophils did not change. Of course, the absolute number of hypodense eosinophils was increased because the total number of eosinophils was increased. What we don't know is whether this means that there is a shift occurring from normal to hypodense and then a replenishment of normal eosinophils.

Wasserman: Two points. First of all, with regard to the economy situation, or the size of the granules. Do we truly know the density of the granules? Are the granules denser than the rest of the cell? They are darker but that doesn't imply density.

Gleich: I don't think we actually know the density of individual granules. We assume, at least I think it is a tacit assumption which no one has really mentioned, that the eosinophil is the densest peripheral granulocyte due to the granules. But I don't think that has been proven.

Wasserman: I'd like to know if the switch from a normodense eosinophil to a hypodense eosinophil, say under stimulation of PAF, is reversible within an individual cell.

Fukuda: I didn't check that, but when I treated eosinophils with CB 3988, which is a PAF blocker, the increasing volume did not occur.

Kay: Neutrophils behave very similarly to eosinophils in many of these systems. It's very easy to up-regulate neutrophils with a variety of chemotactic factors and show similar shifts in density on discontinuous metrizamide gradients. These cells are better cytotoxic cells and they have increased expression of membrane receptors for IgG and CR1 and CR3. These changes are often seen in transient infections, which again parallels the changes in eosinophils. We also have, like you, clearly shown that PAF can convert normodense cells to hypodense cells with an increase in the percentage of IgE rosetting cells which I think would fit in with thoughts in this area.

Capron: I'm very surprised to see the results about the *in vitro* induction of hypodense cells, because I think it must be very difficult to pass the eosinophils twice on the metrizamide gradient; the first time to purify the cells because you start with normodense, and the second time to assess the change in density. I'm very surprised by these results and I think Dr Spry agrees with me, because we have seen that one passage on the metrizamide gradient is able to induce artifactual changes such as cytoplasmic vacuoles. But it has also been shown in the paper by Austen's group, so you are not the only one. My question is related to the changes in density of eosinophils after corticosteroid therapy. You presented results showing a decrease in the proportion of hypodense after corticosteroid therapy in asthmatic patients. In our experiments with Dr Prin with patients with the hypereosinophilic syndrome we have seen an increase in the proportion of hypodense eosinophils after corticosteroid therapy. We have the impression that the normodense population is disappearing after this therapy and now have some evidence that the hypodense populations are corticosteroid resistant. So can you answer that point?

Fukuda: When I performed experiments on *in vitro* induction of hypodense eosinophils, I first obtained leukocyte-rich plasma, then divided it into many aliquots. We then incubated the leukocyte-rich plasma with the ECF-A peptide, PAF or buffer. Finally, the leukocyte rich plasma was fractionated on the gradient.

Capron: So the induction is done on unpurified cells?

Fukuda: Yes.

Gleich: I'm not sure that it came out of Dr Fukuda's presentation but, in fact, on the studies on the patients with hypereosinophilia, the blood was actually taken and divided immediately, so that one fraction was utilized to determine whether or not they indeed were hypodense. And a second fraction was immediately treated to obtain the leukocytes by dextran sedimentation and these were immediately fixed. In other words, there was minimal *in vitro* manipulation to avoid the possibility of being misled by artifact. And the question which should be easy to answer amongst patients who have chronic asthma following exposure to allergens, but perhaps more interestingly amongst patients with idiopathic asthma is: does the severity of the asthma as measured by FEV_1 or some other measure of pulmonary function vary in concert with the number of hypodense eosinophils? I think that's an intriguing question which, I must confess, I'd be most curious about.

Venge: Just a comment to Dr Wasserman about the density of the granules. As I will show in my talk, the granules are much denser than the cells.

Spry: Did you see an excess of lipid bodies in any of the cells which you stimulated with any of these chemicals?

Fukuda: No, I didn't.

Vargaftig: Dr Vadas was looking so sad, you can take 30 seconds.

Vadas: I professionally look sad all the time. Actually, I think you will be sorry . . . As I was sitting here, I asked myself, are we talking about cell density without any of us being real professionals in the field. I don't think we have a real understanding of what determines cell density; for example, the volume of hydration of a cell is much greater than the actual cellular volume that you see. Measuring heterogenous responses induced by ten agents and then trying to make sense of it seems to me to be very hopeful.

Vargaftig: That was a very good way of closing the discussion.

10

Eosinophil Biochemistry and Killing Mechanisms

P. Venge and C. G. B. Peterson

The Laboratory for Inflammation Research,
Department of Clinical Chemistry,
University Hospital, S-751 85 Uppsala, Sweden

10.1 INTRODUCTION

Since its discovery in 1879 by Paul Ehrlich, a role for the eosinophil granulocyte in the defence against parasites has been proposed by several investigators. The role played by the eosinophil in this defence, however, has remained enigmatic, although a direct killing of the parasite by the eosinophil has been suggested. The proposal of a capacity to kill parasites would imply that the eosinophil is capable of tissue destruction. In spite of this it was almost 100 years before the hypothesis was put forward that this putative destructive capability of the eosinophil in some situations might also be turned towards the host (1, 2).

Since this hypothesis has been launched a number of reports have given support to this idea and, indeed, established the eosinophil as a true inflam-

Eosinophils in Asthma
ISBN 0-12-506452-7

Table 1   The major proteins of human eosinophil granules

Protein	Molecular weight (kD)
Eosinophil cationic protein (ECP)	18.5–22
Eosinophil peroxidase (EPO)	67
Eosinophil protein-X (EPX) or eosinophil derived neurotoxin	
(EDN)	23
Major basic protein (MBP)	9.2

matory cell with both pro-inflammatory and probably anti-inflammatory capacities. The basis for the hypothesis of the eosinophil being a destructive cell was the discovery and purification of several highly cationic proteins (3, 4) from the granules of the human eosinophils and the demonstration of the eosinophil as a very potent producer of toxic oxygen metabolites (5). Also, the recognition of the hypereosinophilic syndrome as a clinical entity presenting itself as a disease with a wide variety of serious symptoms (6), probably directly caused by the presence of the great number of eosinophils, has been important in establishing this new view on the eosinophil.

10.2   THE CYTOTOXIC GRANULE PROTEINS OF HUMAN EOSINOPHILS

The protein content of the human eosinophil is dominated by the presence of four major proteins, as depicted in Table 1. For detailed information of their molecular characteristics and biological functions the reader is referred to some recent reviews (7, 8).

The major characteristics of these four proteins are their high isoelectric points, for some of them above pH 11. The first proteins to be purified were ECP and MBP. ECP was originally purified from myeloid cells of chronic myeloid leukaemia patients (9) and termed component 5 of the cationic proteins of human granulocytes and at that time believed to belong to the family of bactericidal proteins of neutrophils. The eosinophil origin of component 5 was not revealed until later (3). MBP was originally purified from guinea-pig eosinophils (10) and later also identified in human eosinophils (4) through the antigenic cross-reactivity between guinea-pig and human MBP. Human MBP was purified from patients with the hypereosinophilic syndrome and in these cells MBP was the clearly dominating granule protein with ECP-concentrations at only 3–15% of the content of normal cells (11). In contrast, in normal eosinophils ECP seems to be one of the dominating proteins with an estimated average content of 26 μg/10^6 cells (12). What these large relative differences in content of hypereosinophilic and normal eosinophils of the two proteins actually reflect is at present uncertain, but may be the heterogeneity of the eosinophils. ECP recently was purified from normal eosinophils and shown to have physicochemical characteristics probably indistinguishable from ECP purified from hypereosinophilic eosinophils and myeloid cells (13). Thus ECP from normal cells is made up by three antigenically related forms with molecular weights from 18.5 to 22 kD. The three forms have identical N-terminal amino acid sequences and amino acid compositions, which in turn are almost identical to those described previously (14, 15). Also the heterogeneity of normal ECP is most likely due to differences in carbohydrate content as has been shown for hypereosinophilic ECP (14).

EPX was purified from both normal and hypereosinophilic eosinophils and shown to be identical (16). Collaborative studies have shown that EPX most likely is identical to EDN both having RNAase activity, molecular weights between 18 and 19 kD after reduction and antigenically closely related (17).

EPO has been purified from both normal and hypereosinophilic eosinophils (18, 19). EPO is a two-chained protein with a heavy chain of 52 kD and a light chain of 15 kD. On purified agarose, EPO migrates to the same position as ECP indicating a very high isoelectric point, i.e. above pH 11 (19). Interestingly EPO is specifically bound to a component in the neutrophil membrane (20).

Human MBP is a 9.2 kD protein which has a strong tendency to polymerize (4). Probably MBP makes up the typical crystalloid structures found in the specific granules of eosinophils. MBP is not entirely specific to the eosinophil since it is also found at low concentrations in such cells as the basophil (21). The cellular content of MBP in normal cells is estimated to be about 5 μg/10^6 cells. This does not necessarily mean that the MBP content is only one-fifth of the ECP of normal cells since different methods have been used in the estimation of the contents of the two proteins. However, these data and the data cited above emphasize that normal eosinophils are quite different from hypereosinophilic eosinophils with respect to granule content.

10.3   GRANULE POPULATIONS AND SECRETION OF PROTEINS

Two populations of granules can be distinguished morphologically in human eosinophils. One is the large, crystalloid containing population which is also

Table 2   Granule populations of normal human eosinophils

Main population	Relative density	Protein content
Peroxidase-positive	Very dense	EPO, MBP ECP, EPX
Peroxidase-negative	Dense	ECP, EPX
	Light	ECP, EPX

peroxidase positive and the other is made up by small peroxidase negative granules. As indicated above the crystalloid structure is probably made up by MBP. By immunohistochemical methods ECP and EPO were shown to be contained in the large crystalloid containing granules (22). In addition, ECP was observed in the small peroxidase-negative granules. Separation of normal eosinophil granules on a sucrose density gradient revealed at least 4 peaks containing eosinophil proteins (23). One heavy peak at an equilibrium density of 1.248 g/ml which contained all EPO and approximately 40% of respectively ECP and EPX. Two light peaks at 1.211 and 1.229 g/ml which contained no EPO but which together contained approximately 40% of ECP and 30% of EPX. One very light peak, coinciding with the membrane fraction, contained no EPO but approximately 10% of ECP and 20% of EPX. As indicated in Table 2 we conclude from these data and the data of others that the granules of human eosinophils are made up by two distinctive populations one peroxidase-negative and one peroxidase-positive of which the peroxidase-negative may be present in more than one subpopulation.

Previous investigations have shown that optimal ECP release from human eosinophils is achieved when the cells are exposed to particles such as Sephadex G-15, coated with serum proteins, presumably C3b (24). Others have demonstrated peroxidase and MBP release but no ECP release after exposure of hypodense cells to IgE complexes in contrast to the release of ECP which occurred when the eosinophils were exposed to IgG complexes (25). These data suggest that eosinophil granule proteins may be released differentially from the cell dependent upon the stimulus to which the cell is exposed and dependent upon the state of activity of the cell. The latter was because hypodense eosinophils in many respects, such as parasite killing, production of oxidative metabolites etc., have been shown to be more active than normodense cells (26).

To study the mechanisms of release of eosinophil granule proteins in more detail a number of experiments have been initiated in which the simultaneous measurement of the three granule proteins ECP, EPX and EPO is made by radioimmunoassay (23). With Sephadex G-15 particles coated with serum proteins the release of ECP and EPX from normal eosinophils was exactly identical, both the kinetics and the quantity, irrespective of pretreatment of the particles, i.e. washed, unwashed or unopsonized. Maximum release of both ECP and EPX was approximately 20% of total after 60 minutes with particles in the presence of serum. This release was contrasted by a complete absence of detectable EPO in the supernatant. In another set of experiments the glyceride, IpOCOC$_9$, was used since this glyceride in other experiments had initiated a significant release of ECP in contrast to the phorbolester PMA (24, unpublished observation). IpOCOC$_9$ has been shown to degranulate human basophils non-cytotoxically by means of protein kinase C activation and by a hyperosmolar mechanism. IpOCOC$_9$ induced a release of about 40% of EPX in contrast to the release of only 10% of ECP. Also, release of EPO was detected in these experiments but only to a degree of 3–5% of the total cellular content. These data support the view that the granule proteins of eosinophils may be released selectively, although they are contained in the same granule population. This could also mean that different transduction signals are involved in the government of the release of the different granule proteins.

10.4   THE CYTOTOXIC ACTIVITIES OF EOSINOPHIL GRANULE PROTEINS

One of the most conspicuous features of the four granule proteins is their capacity to cause injury to both mammalian and non-mammalian cells.

Both ECP, EPO and MBP kill the schistosomula of *Schistosoma mansoni in vitro* (27–30). EPO-mediated killing needs the presence of H$_2$O$_2$ and a halide to kill efficiently schistosomula. H$_2$O$_2$ is one of the products formed during activation of the eosinophil in contact with an opsonized parasite which makes this mechanism a likely killing mechanism *in vivo* as well. The killing of schistosomula by ECP occurred at lower concentrations than with MBP indicating that ECP on a molar basis is more cytotoxic than MBP (31). If instead lung-stage larvae of *Schistosoma mansoni* were used as target organisms ECP was almost without any effect. This was contrasted by EPX since this protein, which was without any effects on the schistosomula, actually quite efficiently killed the lung-stage larvae. The reason for these differences in cytotoxic activities towards the two different forms of *Schistosomula mansoni* is not known but indicates that the mode of action of ECP and EPX with respect to parasite killing is different. EPO and MBP were also shown to kill other parasites such as *T. cruzi* and *T. spiralis* (32–34).

10.4.1   Nervous Tissue

The development of ataxia and other CNS symptoms was described by Gordon after the injection of extracts of lymph node material from Hodgkin patients into the brain ventricles of rabbits (35). The most conspicuous histological finding was the destruction of the Purkinje cells of the cerebellum. The phenomenon was termed the "Gordon phenomenon". Subsequent findings suggested that the neurotoxic effect was related to the number of eosinophils present in the extract (36). Attempts were, therefore, made to define the neurotoxic agent of the eosinophils. The protein thus identified was purified and termed eosinophil derived neurotoxin (EDN) (see above) (37). In other experiments the purified proteins ECP and EPX were injected into the ventricles of the brains of experimental animals (38). These experiments showed that both proteins were capable of producing the Gordon phenomenon and the typical histological picture. However, in these experiments ECP was about 100 times more potent and induced the Gordon phenomenon within some weeks after injection of as little as 60 ng of protein. Although potent, it was also suggested that the effects of these granule proteins are quite unspecific and unselective since they would destroy any cell or structure dependent on the deposition of the material (39).

In a patient with achalasia of oesophagus secondary to gastric cancer a massive infiltration of activated eosinophils was seen in the muscularis of the oesophagus with signs of secretion of large amounts of ECP. In contrast a nearly total absence of the neurotransmitters VIP, substance-P and AChE was observed (40). This finding further suggests the neurotoxicity of eosinophil granule proteins, notably ECP.

10.4.2   Respiratory Tract

The exposure of epithelial cells to micromolar concentrations of MBP produced extensive damage and a histological picture reminiscent of the pathological changes seen in human bronchial asthma (41). MBP also affects ciliary functions with impairment of ciliary beating. Instillation of small amounts of ECP produced very similar pictures, i.e. with epithelial cell damage and patchy denudation of the epithelial cell layer both in trachea and the bronchi and cell plugging (42). By immunohistochemical techniques both ECP and MBP were demonstrated in the lung tissue of patients dying from asthma (43, 44). The staining suggested extracellular deposition of the proteins indicating degranulation of the eosinophils in the respiratory tract. More direct evidence of secretion of ECP was obtained when elevated levels of ECP were measured in bronchoalveolar lung fluid during the late-asthmatic reaction after allergen inhalation challenge of asthmatic individuals (45).

10.4.3 Intestine

Guinea-pig MBP has been shown to be toxic to intestinal cells (7) and in patients with Crohn's disease eosinophil infiltration has been observed, which suggests a role for the eosinophil (46). Intestinal fluid from the small intestine of patients with Crohn's disease and the adult coeliac disease sometimes contain highly elevated concentrations of ECP when compared to normals (47). Biopsies from the jejunal cell wall of patients with the adult coeliac disease showed a remarkable infiltration of eosinophils in areas with ulceration. When the sections were stained for ECP, the results suggested a heavy extracellular deposition of ECP in these areas indicating active degranulation of the eosinophils. This picture was contrasted by areas of undamaged intestinal wall where eosinophils were also present but where no such extracellular deposition of ECP was observed. These results suggest that the eosinophil had taken part in the processes leading to ulceration of the intestinal wall in adult coeliac disease and that ulceration may be caused by among other things the cytotoxic eosinophil granule proteins.

10.4.4 Other Organs and Cells

Endomyocardial disease is one of the typical clinical findings in patients with hypereosinophilia. Eosinophil cationic proteins were shown to be toxic to heart muscle cells *in vitro* (48) and ECP was demonstrated in the myocardium of patients suffering from myocardial disease (49). The findings were interpreted to indicate a role for the cytotoxic eosinophil granule proteins in such diseases. In other experiments MBP has been shown to be cytotoxic to lymphoma cells and a variety of other mammalian cells (50). The cytotoxicity of ECP was assayed by means of lysis of red blood cells (51). Also, a macrophage cell line was shown to be susceptible to the cytotoxic action of ECP.

Some non-cytotoxic effects of ECP, EPX and MBP are the induction of histamine release from rat mast cells by ECP and MBP and the induction of histamine release from human blood basophils (52, 53). Moreover, ECP and EPX were shown to potently inhibit lymphocyte proliferation after mitogen or antigen stimulation (54). All these non-cytotoxic effects on various cells indicate that the eosinophil by virtue of its granule proteins has the capacity to modify immunological and allergic reactions without necessarily causing damage to the involved cells.

10.4.5   Mechanism of the Cytotoxic Action of Eosinophil Granule Proteins

The above examples clearly suggest that the granule proteins of human eosinophils have the capacity to destroy almost any cell, mammalian or non-mammalian. Attempts were therefore made to study the mechanism of action of these proteins. For these purposes a lipid vesicle-permeability assay was used. By means of this technique it was demonstrated that ECP caused leakiness of the vesicles to monovalent ions and to a certain extent also to divalent ions (51). Further studies with phospholipid planar lipid bilayers showed typical changes in the conductance when exposed to ECP. These changes were indicative of opening of individual channels which became incorporated into the membrane. The channels thus opened were remarkably resistant to closing by high transmembrane voltage in a way very similar to poly-C_9-channels i.e. the channels formed by the complement component C_9. Further experiments indicated that ECP was the dominating pore-forming protein in the granules of human eosinophils with EPX causing leakage by crosslinking membrane structures instead of making pores. Recent ultrastructural studies by Dr Ding-E Young have identified ring-like structures in liposomes which are approximately 50 Å wide (unpublished). This demonstration would thus support the notion of ECP making pores in cellular membranes. It is therefore likely that ECP belongs to the growing family of pore-forming proteins produced by a variety of cells such as cytotoxic T lymphocytes (55).

10.5   INHIBITORS OF EOSINOPHIL GRANULE PROTEINS

It is reasonable to hypothesize that the organism has been provided with principles that antagonize the potent cytotoxic activities of the described eosinophil granule proteins. Thus it has been demonstrated that both ECP and MBP are neutralized by heparin (56, 57). ECP binds to heparin in a 1:1 molar complex (unpublished Dahl & Venge). The question raised to these findings is for obvious reasons their relevance since it would be anticipated that the acid heparin would bind to any basic protein. However, it should be kept in mind that heparin is contained in mast cells and probably released from the mast cells during activation and therefore probably in many situations released in parallel to ECP from the eosinophils in the same reaction.

Another antagonist of ECP of potential interest is α_2-macroglobulin (α_2M) since this molecule very recently has been shown to bind ECP under certain conditions (58). Thus only α_2M that had been briefly exposed to proteases such as cathepsin G or thrombin would bind ECP. Also the exposure of α_2M to methylamine, which is used to inhibit protease binding to α_2M, transformed α_2M into an efficient binder of ECP. These measures are known to change α_2M from the "slow" form to the "fast" form (59). The biological relevance of the binding of ECP to α_2M is suggested by the study of serum of patients with the hypereosinophilic syndrome. In these sera a high molecular weight form of ECP is observed, which indicates that some ECP in this situation is bound to a high molecular weight compound presumably α_2M (60). The fact that similar high molecular weight forms are not found in sera of normal individuals is probably due to a very fast elimination of the protein complex akin to the fast elimination of protease-α_2M complexes (61).

Another finding that may have a bearing on the biological relevance of the α_2M interaction with ECP is the fast reduction of ECP after allergen inhalation challenge of asthmatics (62) and the paradoxically low levels of ECP in severe asthma (63). Although we have not been able directly to demonstrate the production of the "fast" form of α_2M in these situations, we speculate that during the acute asthmatic reaction and during ongoing asthma products are generated which alter α_2M in this direction giving rise to an accelerated ECP-elimination from plasma. After allergen challenge the elimination rate, $t_{\frac{1}{2}}$ for ECP, is less than 15 min whereas normal elimination of ECP is on average 35 min (unpublished observation).

10.6   MEASUREMENT OF EOSINOPHIL GRANULE PROTEINS IN BODY FLUIDS

As described above most of the cytotoxic effects of the eosinophil granule proteins have been observed at concentrations between 10^{-8} and 10^{-6} M which for ECP corresponds to weight concentrations of about 200–20 000 μg/l. Normal concentrations in human serum are in the range from 5 to 55 μg/l (60) and in patients with eosinophilia findings of concentrations up to 20 000 μg/l have been made but are rare. However, in various body fluids, very high levels of ECP have been measured which tell us that the concentrations used *in vitro* to demonstrate various cytotoxic effects of ECP are quite realistic. Similar observations have been made for MBP (7). Below are given some examples of clinical studies in which ECP has been measured and where levels are found which emphasize this statement.

ECP was measured in bronchoalveolar lavage after allergen challenge and elevated levels were found in particular in those individuals who developed a late asthmatic reaction. Maximum concentrations in these fluids were 130 μg/l which probably means that the concentrations in lung lining fluid are 10–100 times higher (45). In nasal fluid concentrations of ECP up to 5000 μg/l were measured (64). In the latter case the true concentrations were estimated by the use of lithium in the washing fluid as internal standard. In a third study of the respiratory tract ECP was measured in the bronchoalveolar lavage fluid in patients with adult respiratory distress syndrome (ARDS) and in these patients levels as high as 300 μg/l were found (65). Thus in, all three studies, ECP levels were observed which are fully comparable with the concentrations of ECP needed in vitro to exert cytotoxic activities on respiratory tract cells.

In a study of patients with various kinds of diseases of the CNS, such as multiple sclerosis, stroke, viral meningitis, supranormal ECP cerebrospinal fluid levels were seen but stayed within the range of 20 μg/l and below (66). However, in three patients with bacterial meningitis and a very poor clinical outcome, ECP levels up to 500 μg/l were found. This observation certainly does not prove a causal relationship between ECP-levels and the central nervous symptoms but is intriguing since equivalent to 100 μg/l ECP in the cerebrospinal fluid of a rabbit produced severe CNS symptoms within a couple of weeks.

10.7 CONCLUSION

The human eosinophil is armed with a number of very potent cytotoxic granule proteins which upon extracellular release may produce considerable damage. As indicated in Figure 1 these proteins have cytotoxic properties of their own but in combination with cytotoxic oxygen metabolites the cytotoxicity may be considerably enhanced (67). The toxic effect of the proteins seems to be quite unselective and affect most mammalian and non-mammalian cells. It is likely that these toxic principles are meant to protect the organism from invading organisms such as parasites. However, when released uncontrolled in the organism they may participate in the production of diseases such as asthma, the adult coeliac disease etc. The protection towards the action of the proteins therefore seems vital and the discovery of α_2-macroglobulin as a specific binder of ECP may be relevant in this regard.

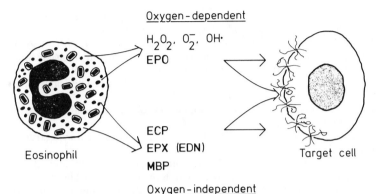

Oxygen-dependent

H_2O_2, O_2^-, OH·
EPO

ECP
EPX (EDN)
MBP

Eosinophil

Target cell

Oxygen-independent

Fig. 1 The killing mechanisms of the human eosinophil granulocyte. The figure intends to illustrate the fact that both oxygen-dependent and independent mechanisms are operative in killing of target cells. Presumably these two principles work together in a synergistic way.

Finally, however, it should be emphasized that the eosinophil may have other important physiological roles other than, for example, the damage of parasites. Thus the demonstration of regulatory properties of ECP and EPX on immunological reactions and of ECP on certain aspects of the coagulation cascade (68) and fibrinolysis (69), in addition to the demonstration of effects of eosinophil material on fibroblast growth (70), certainly support this notion.

Acknowledgement

Part of the work cited in this review was supported by grants from the Swedish Medical Research Council and the Swedish Board of Technical Development.

REFERENCES

1. Spry, C. J. F. and Tai, P. C. (1976). Studies on blood eosinophils II. Patients with Löffler's cardiomyopathy. *Clin. Exp. Immunol.* **24**, 423–434.
2. Olsson, I. and Venge, P. (1979). The role of the eosinophil granulocyte in the inflammatory reaction. *Allergy* **34**, 353–367.
3. Gleich, G. J., Loegering, D. A., Mann, K. G. and Maldonado, J. E. (1976). Com-

parative properties of the Charcot–Leyden crystal protein and the major basic protein from human eosinophils. *J. Clin. Invest.* **57**, 633–640.

4. Olsson, I., Venge, P., Spitznagel, J. K. and Lehrer, R.I. (1977). Arginine-rich cationic proteins of human eosinophil granules. Comparison of the constituents of eosinophilic and neutrophilic leukocytes. *Lab. Invest.* **36**, 493–500.

5. Baehner, R. L. and Johnston, R. B. (1971). Metabolic and bactericidal activities of human eosinophils. *Br. J. Haematol.* **20**, 277–285.

6. Spry, C. J. F. (1982). The hypereosinophilic syndrome: Clinical features, laboratory findings and treatment. *Allergy* **37**, 539–51.

7. Gleich, G. J. and Adolphson, C. R. (1986). The eosinophil leukocyte: structure and function. *Adv. Immunol.* **39**, 177–253.

8. Venge, P. (1985). The eosinophil in inflammation. In: "Inflammation" (Eds P. Venge, and A. Lindbom), 85–103. Almqvist & Wiksell, Stockholm.

9. Olsson, I. and Venge, P. (1974). Cationic proteins of human granulocytes. II. Separation of the cationic proteins of the granules of leukemic myeloid cells. *Blood* **44**, 235–246.

10. Gleich, G. J., Loegering, D. A. and Maldonado, J. E. (1973). Identification of a major basic protein in guinea pig eosinophil granules. *J. Exp. Med.* **173**, 1459–1471.

11. Ackerman, S. J., Loegering, D. A., Venge, P., Olsson, I., Harley, J. B., Fauci, A. S. and Gleich, G. J. (1983). Distinctive cationic proteins of the human eosinophil granule: Major basic protein, eosinophil cationic protein, and eosinophil derived neurotoxin. *J. Immunol.* **131**, 2977–2982.

12. Dahl, R., Venge, P. and Olsson, I. (1978). The content of eosinophil cationic protein in eosinophil leucocytes. Study on normal controls and patients with bronchial asthma. *Allergy* **33**, 152–154.

13. Peterson, C. G. B., Jörnvall, H. and Venge, P. (1988). Purification and characterization of eosinophil cationic protein from norma human eosinophils. *Eur. J. Haematol* **40**, 415–420.

14. Gleich, G. J., Loegering, D. A., Bell, M. P., Chekel, J. L., Ackerman, S. J. and McKean, D. J. (1986). Biochemical and functional similarities between human eosinophil-derived neurotoxin and eosinophil cationic protein: Homology with ribonuclease. *Proc. Natl. Acad. Sci. USA* **83**, 3146–3150.

15. Olsson, I., Persson, A-M. and Winqvist, I. (1986). Biochemical properties of the eosinophil cationic protein and demonstration of its biosynthesis *in vitro* in marrow cells from patients with an eosinophilia. *Blood* **67**, 498–503.

16. Peterson, C. G. B. and Venge, P. (1983). Purification and characterization of a new cationic protein—eosinophil protein-X (EPX)—from granules of human eosinophils. *Immunology* **50**, 19–26.

17. Slifman, N. R., Peterson, C. G. B., Gleich, G. J., Dunnette, S. L. and Venge, P. Eosinophil derived neurotoxin and eosinophil protein-x: Comparison of physicochemical, immunologic, and enzymatic properties. (Submitted for publication)

18. Olsen, R. L. and Little, C. (1983). Purification and some properties of myeloperoxidase and eosinophil peroxidase from human blood. *Biochem. J.* **209**, 781–787.

19. Carlson, M. G. Ch., Peterson, C. G. B. and Venge, P. (1985). Human eosinophil peroxidase: Purification and characterization. *J. Immunol.* **134**, 1875–1879.

20. Zabucchi, G., Menegazzi, R., Soranzo, M. R. and Patriarca, (1986). Binding and inactivation sites for eosinophil peroxidase on human eosinophils. *Am. J. Pathol.* **124**, 510–518.

21. Ackerman, S. J., Kephart, G. M., Habermann, T. M., Greipp, P. R. and Gleich, G. J. (1983). Localization of eosinophil granule major basic protein in human basophils. *J. Exp. Med.* **158**, 946–961.
22. Egesten, A., Alumets, J., von Mecklenburg, C., Palmegren, M. and Olsson, I. (1986). Localization of eosinophil cationic protein, major basic protein, and eosinophil peroxidase in human eosinophils by immunoelectron microscopic technique. *J. Histochem. Cytochem.* **34**, 1399–1403.
23. Peterson, C. G. B., Garcia, R. C., Carlson, M. G. C. and Venge, P. Eosinophil cationic protein (ECP), eosinophil protein x (EPX) and eosinophil peroxidase (EPO): Granule distribution, degranulation and characterization of released proteins. (Submitted for publication)
24. Winqvist, I., Olofsson, T. and Olsson, I. (1984). Mechanisms for eosinophil degranulation; release of the eosinophil cationic protein. *Immunol.* **51**, 1–8.
25. Capron, M. and Capron, A. (1987). The IgE receptor of human eosinophils. *In* "Allergy and Inflammation" (Ed. A. B. Kay), 151–159. Academic Press, London.
26. Pincus, S. H., Schooley, W. R., DiNapoli, A. M. and Broder, S. (1981). Metabolic heterogeneity of eosinophils from normal and hypereosinophilic patients. *Blood* **58**, 1175–1181.
27. Butterworth, A. E., Wasson, D. L., Gleich, G. J., Loegering, D. A. and David, J. R. (1979). Damage to schistosomula of Schistosoma mansoni induced directly by eosinophil major basic protein. *J. Immunol.* **122**, 221–229.
28. McLaren, D. J., McKean, J. R., Olsson, I., Venge, P. and Kay, A. B. (1981). Morphological studies on the killing of schistosomula of Schistosoma mansoni by human eosinophil and neutrophil cationic proteins *in vitro*. *Parasite Immunol.* **3**, 359–373.
29. Jong, E. C., Mahmoud, A. A. F. and Klebanoff, S. J. (1981). Peroxidase mediated toxicity to schistosomula of Schistosoma mansoni. *J. Immunol.* **126**, 468–471.
30. McLaren, D. J., Peterson, C. G. B. and Venge, P. (1984). Schistosoma mansoni: further studies of the interaction between schistosomula and granulocyte-derived cationic proteins *in vitro*. *Parasitology* **88**, 491–503.
31. Ackerman, S. J., Gleich, G. J., Loegering, D. A., Richardson, B. A. and Butterworth, A. E. (1985). Comparative toxicity of purified human eosinophil granule cationic proteins for schistosomula of *Schistosoma mansoni*. *Am. J. Trop. Med. Hyg.* **34**, 735–745.
32. Wassom, D. L. and Gleich, G. J. (1979). Damage to *Trichinella spiralis* newborn larvae by eosinophil major basic protein. *Am. J. Trop. Med. Hyg.* **28**, 860–863.
33. Kierszenbaum, F., Ackerman, S. J. and Gleich, G. J. Destruction of bloodstream forms of *Trypanosoma cruzi* by eosinophil granule major basic protein. *Am. J. Trop. Med. Hyg.* **30**, 775–779.
34. Buys, J., Wever, R. and Ruitenberg, E. J. (1984). Myeloperoxidase is more efficient than eosinophil peroxidase in the *in vitro* killing of newborn larvae of *Trichinella spiralis*. *Immunology* **51**, 601–607.
35. Gordon, M. H. (1932). "Studies of the Aetiology of Lymphadenoma", 7–76. John Wright, Bristol.
36. Durack, D. T., Sumi, S. M. and Klebanoff, S. J. (1979). Neurotoxicity of human eosinophils. *Proc. Natl. Acad. Sci. USA* **76**, 1443–1447.
37. Durack, D. T., Ackerman, S. J., Loegering, D. A. and Gleich, G. J. (1981). Purification of eosinophil-derived neurotoxin. *Proc. Natl. Acad. Sci. USA* **78**, 5165–5169.
38. Fredens, K., Dahl, R. and Venge, P. (1982). The Gordon phenomenon induced by

the eosinophil cationic protein and eosinophil protein x. *J. Allergy Clin. Immunol.* **70**, 361–366.

39. Fredens, K., Dahl, R. and Venge, P. (1985). Eosinophils and cellular injury. *NER Allergy Proc.* **6**, 346–351.

40. Fredens, K., Tottrup, A., Kristensen Bayer, I., Dahl, R., Jacobsen, N. O., Funch-Jensen, P. and Thommesen, P. Severe destruction of esophageal nerves in a patient with achalasia secondary to gastric cancer. A possible role of eosinophil neurotoxic proteins. *Digest Dis. Sci.* (In press).

41. Frigas, E., Loegering, D. A. and Gleich, G. J. (1980). Cytotoxic effects of the guinea pig eosinophil major basic protein in tracheal epithelium. *Lab. Invest.* **42**, 35–43.

42. Dahl, R., Fredens, K., Marcussen, C. and Venge, P. (1985). Eosinophils and bronchial injury. *Ann. Meet. Eur. Acad. Allergol. Clin. Immunol.* **Abstr. 63976**.

43. Filley, W. V., Holley, K. E., Kephart, G. M. and Gleich, G. J. (1982). Identification by immunofluorescence of eosinophil granule major basic protein in lung tissues of patients with bronchial asthma. *Lancet* **2**, 11–16.

44. Dahl, R., Venge, P. and Fredens, K. (1988). The eosinophil. *In* "Asthma: Basic Mechanisms and Clinical Management" (Eds P. J. Barnes, I. Rodger and N. Thomson), 115–129. Academic Press, London.

45. DeMonchy, J. G. R., Kauffman, H. F., Venge, P., Koeter, G. H., Jansen, H. M., Sluiter, H. J., DeVries, K. (1985). Bronchoalveolar eosinophilia during allergen-induced late asthmatic reactions. *Am. Rev. Respir. Dis.* **131**, 373–376.

46. Dvorak, A. M. (1980). Ultrastructural evidence for release of major basic protein-containing crystalline cores of eosinophil granules *in vivo*: Cytotoxic potential in Crohn's disease. *J. Immunol.* **125**, 460–462.

47. Hällgren, R., Colombel, J. F., Dahl, R., Fredens, K., Kruse, A., Jacobsen, S., Venge, P. and Rambaud, J. C. (1989). Neutrophil and eosinophil involvement of the small bowel in patients with celiac disease and Crohn's disease. Studies on the secretion rate and immunohistochemical localization of granulocyte granule constituents in jejunum. *Ann. J. Med.* **86**, 56–64.

48. Tai, P-C., Hayes, D. J., Clark, J. B. and Spry, C. J. F. (1982). Toxic effects of human eosinophil secretion products on isolated rat heart cells *in vitro*. *Biochem. J.* **204**, 75–80.

49. Spry, C. J. F., Tai, P-C., Davies, J. (1983). The cardiotoxicity of eosinophils. *Postgrad. Med. J.* **59**, 147–151.

50. Gleich, G. J., Frigas, E., Loegering, D. A., Wassom, D. L. and Steinmuller, D. (1979). Cytotoxic properties of the eosinophil major basic protein. *J. Immunol.* **123**, 2925–2927.

51. Ding-E. Young, J., Peterson, C. G. B., Venge, P. and Cohn, Z. A. (1986). Mechanism of membrane damage mediated by human eosinophil cationic protein. *Nature* **321**, 613–616.

52. O'Donnell, M. G., Ackerman, S. J., Gleich, G. J. and Thomas, L. L. Activation of basophil and mast cell histamine release by eosinophil granule major basic protein. *J. Exp. Med.* **157**, 1981–1991.

53. Bergstrand, H., Lundquist, B., Peterson, B.Á., Peterson, C. and Venge, P. (1985). Eosinophil derived cationic proteins and human leukocyte histamine release. In: "Inflammation" (Eds P. Venge and A. Lindbom), 361–366. Almqvist & Wiksell, Stockholm.

54. Peterson, C. G. B., Skoog, V. and Venge, P. (1986). Human eosinophil cationic

proteins (ECP and EPX) and their suppressive effects on lymphocyte proliferation. *Immunobiol.* **171**, 1–3.

55. Ding-E Young, J. (1985). Cytolytic proteins. In "Inflammation" (Eds P. Venge, A. Lindbom), 329–340. Almqvist & Wiksell, Stockholm.

56. Gleich, G. J., Loegering, D. A., Frigas, E., Wassom, D. L., Solley, G. O. and Mann, K. G. (1980). The major basic protein of the eosinophil granule: Physicochemical properties, localization, and function. *In* "The Eosinophil in Health and Disease" (Eds A. A. F. Mahmoud, K. F. Austen), 79–94. Grune Stratton, New York.

57. Venge, P., Dahl, R., Fredens, K., Hällgren, R. and Peterson, C. (1983). Eosinophil cationic proteins (ECP and EPX) in health and disease. *In* "Immunobiology of the Eosinophil" (Eds T. Yoshida, M. Torisu), 163–179. Elsevier, New York.

58. Peterson, C. G. B. and Venge, P. (1987). Interaction and complex-formation between the eosinophil cationic protein and α_2-macroglobulin. *Biochem. J.* **245**, 781–787.

59. Barrett, A. J., Brown, M. A. and Sayers, C. A. (1979). The electrophoretically "slow" and "fast" forms of the α_2-macroglobulin molecule. *Biochem. J.* **181**, 401–418.

60. Venge, P., Roxin, L-E. and Olsson, I. (1977). Radioimmunoassay of human eosinophil cationic protein. *Br. J. Haematol.* **37**, 331–335.

61. Ohlsson, K. and Laurell, C. B. (1976). The disappearance of enzyme-inhibitor complexes from the circulation of man. *Clin. Sci. Mol. Med.* **51**, 87–93.

62. Dahl, R., Venge, P. and Olsson, I. (1978). Variations of blood eosinophils and eosinophil cationic protein in serum in patients with bronchial asthma: studies during inhalation challenge test. *Allergy* **33**, 211–215.

63. Venge, P., Zetterström, O., Dahl, R., Roxin, L.-E. and Olsson, I. (1977). Low levels of eosinophil cationic proteins in patients with asthma. *Lancet* **8034**, 373–375.

64. Linder, A., Venge, P. and Deuschl, H. (1987). Eosinophil cationic protein and myeloperoxidase in nasal secretion as markers of inflammation in allergic rhinitis. *Allergy* **42**, 583–590.

65. Hällgren, R., Samuelsson, T., Venge, P. and Modig, J. (1987). Eosinophil activation in the lung is related to lung damage in adult respiratory distress syndrome. *Am. Rev. Resp. Dis.* **135**, 639–642.

66. Hällgren, R., Terent, A. and Venge, P. (1983). Eosinophil cationic protein (ECP) in the cerebrospinal fluid. *J. Neurol. Sci.* **58**, 57–71.

67. Yazdanbakhsh, M., Tai, P. C., Spry, C. J. F., Gleich, G. J. and Roos, D. (1987). Synergism between eosinophil cationic protein and oxygen metabolites in killing of schistosomula of *Schistosoma mansoni*. *J. Immunol.* **138**, 3443–3447.

68. Venge, P., Dahl, R. and Hällgren, R. (1979). Enhancement of factor XII dependent reactions by eosinophil cationic protein. *Thromb. Res.* **14**, 641–649.

69. Dahl, R. and Venge, P. (1979). Enhancement of urokinase-induced plasminogen activation by the cationic protein of human eosinophil granulocytes. *Thromb. Res.* **14**, 599–608.

70. Pincus, S. H., Ramesh, K. S. and Wyler, D. J. (1987). Eosinophils stimulate fibroblast DNA synthesis. *Blood* **70**, 572–574.

DISCUSSION

Vargaftig (Chairman)

Gleich: One has to be very cautious, at least in the case of EDN, about making conclusions regarding whether or not the level that you measure in fact derives from eosinophils. The same holds incidently for MBP. MBP is produced by placental X cells and likely by placental giant cells. The function of these cells is of course totally obscure. In collaboration with Dr Don Glitz who is professor of Biochemistry at the University of California, L.A., we have been able to compare data with him indicating that (EDN) EPX is identical to human liver ribonuclease which has now been completely sequenced. These sources outside the eosinophil and the sticky nature of these proteins make conclusions about differential secretion hazardous.

Venge: Maybe I should take the point of differential secretion. You are absolutely right. And for this reason we today do it the other way around. We stimulate the cells and then we subfractionate the granules and then we look at what's left in these various granule populations of the proteins, which may be a more correct way to show this phenomenon. So, we'll see if we end up with the same conclusion. I was very intrigued to hear about the liver ribonuclease. Is it an antigenically related protein as well? I mean, is EPX (EDN) from the eosinophils antigenically related to the ribonuclease in the liver?

Gleich: We actually haven't studied the antigenic relationships, but the amino acid sequence up to residue 60 is identical.

Venge: But you don't know if the antibodies pick up this in your assay?

Gleich: I'd be a monkey's uncle if they don't.

Capron: I was interested in your first slide, to see the existence of peroxidase positive and peroxidase negative granules. Do you mean that the composition of individual granules inside the same eosinophil can be different?

Venge: Yes, I think so and I think this is what Juge Olsson and his group showed. They showed, if I remember correctly, in the same eosinophil, that EPO was present in the same granules as ECP but there were other granules which only had ECP inside, and not EPO.

Capron: So we can speculate that in the case of eosinophils from patients, you might have differences in the expression of such granules with less or more EPO.

Venge: Certainly, and that is what we are investigating right now.

Capron: And the second question is related to the neurotoxin. Is it true that the clear demonstration of the neurotoxicity of these substances has been only shown in a heterologous situation by injection of human ECP into an animal species, or has somebody shown that ECP from a given animal is also able to induce a neurotoxic syndrome in the same species?

Venge: I still think it's true that we have been using human ECP, (EDN) EPX and injecting it into animals. I don't know of any species with a homologous system. Do you know Jerry?

Gleich: No, I don't know. I'm not aware, in agreement with what you say, that in fact EDN or EPX or ECP when injected into your or my cerebrospinal fluid, God forbid, would actually cause a neurotoxic reaction. I wouldn't be surprised, but I don't know of any data that force one to that belief at the present time. The second point is that your experiments showing that ECP was exceedingly neurotoxic and about 100 times more active than EPX (EDN), were done in guinea-pigs. Our experiments were done in rabbits. And in doing those titrations à la protocol that Klebanoff and his colleagues did some years ago, we were not able to show this hundredfold molar difference. But we did it in rabbits and you did it in guinea-pigs and that could well be a species difference. In some recent experiments utilizing neuronal development *in vitro*, we found that if you take all the four granule proteins and put them in with developing neurons, and this was done by a colleague in neurology, we observed that (EDN) EPX and ECP inhibited the neuronal development whereas MBP and EPO did not.

Venge: There is another point about this as well. As I suggested in my talk, we know today that there is heterogeneity in activity of ECPs. Some ECPs are quite inactive in any respect and some ECP preparations are very active. This also is an important point to consider.

Dahl: I have a comment on the differential secretions. We looked at it in another way on histology sections of different tissues with eosinophilia, where we see eosinophil degranulation and tissue and destruction. On tissue from the cystitic bladder, there was secretion only of EPX, very little ECP was secreted. As to neurotoxicity in the human situation, in about 30 patients with achalasia we have some specimens from the oesophagus and they are always heavily infiltrated with eosinophils. The eosinophils infiltrate around the ganglion of the Auerbach plexus and destroy it. In those situations we can't detect substance-P or acetylcholine. The autonomic nervous system seems to be out of function or the mediators are not present. So, I think it's some evidence that we have effects of these proteins on nervous tissue and nervous control in human disease. Maybe the same thing will be able to be shown in the bronchi. I'd like to ask you if there have been studies on the killing mechanism of EPO and that these killing mechanisms towards parasites are enhanced if you mix EPO with mast cell granules? What is it in mast cell granules that enhances the EPO killing?

Venge: Actually I don't know, but I know that the peroxidase activity of EPO will be enhanced by whatever surface it's bound to.

Dahl: No, but it could be because mast cells are often seen in connection with eosinophilia in tissues.

Venge: Yes. I have no idea about the mechanism.

Bruijnzeel: Could you explain to me, and perhaps Professor Gleich could as well, how eosinophils in asthma or eczema are being triggered in the *in vivo* situation? Which factor triggers them? Everyone is speaking about the release of a lot of mediators, but I think you first have to find the first trigger.

Venge: Well, that's a difficult point to speculate about. In our hands, the system of using a particle opsonized with serum, and this is presumably C3b, is a very good trigger and I think this could very likely happen *in vivo* as well.

Gleich: I would like to make a comment about the occurrence of eosinophil granule proteins in mast cells. First of all, there is a series of observations which come out of Ann Dvorak's laboratory where she found variable peroxidase positivity in basophil granules, and in an experiment which she did in conjunction with Seymour Klebanoff, showed very clearly that the horse eosinophil peroxidase could be endocytosed and stored in guinea-pig basophils. In recent experiments we have found MBP clearly localized in mast cell granules from human tissues. And in addition to that, we have a mast cell leukaemia cell line which Dr Joseph Butterfield has isolated from a patient with mast cell leukaemia that makes MBP, leading us to the hypothesis that mast cells make MBP. Now, in experiments to address that question, we have been led to an alternative hypothesis that, like the basophils' ability to take up EPO, the mast cell has the ability to take up MBP. The MBP positivity of mast cells probably does not reside in their ability to synthesize the molecule, although that could happen in a leukaemic cell, but rather in their ability to endocytose and to store the molecule in their heparin containing granules.

Vargaftig: Might heparin-like substances devoid of important anti-coagulant effects have anti-asthmatic effects?

Venge: Maybe so, I don't know.

Kay: It was very interesting to see such very high levels of ECP in nasal washes. Was this associated with gross epithelial damage as you might expect?

Venge: This was not looked for in these experiments, but it is something we are going to look at more carefully.

Vadas: Not an answer but a comment on Dr Bruijnzeel's question which obviously is a very important one. We certainly do know that in inflammatory sites, like joints and cavities, where there are inflammatory cells, there are large concentrations of growth factors like GM-CSF and also large concentrations of tumour necrosis factor; so, you have to consider that these cells exist in a different macro-environment than they exist in the blood and then you have to be cogniscant of how the physiology of these cells alters. Neutrophils, after seeing tumour necrosis factor, start to recognize particles which they totally ignored before, like unopsonized zymosan. So, with eosinophils it may be the same. Things that you don't imagine are triggers for degranulation, mucous or bare epithelial surface, may be very powerful triggers, provided they are in the right micro-environment.

Gleich: A comment relating to the development of eosinophils. Judah Denver with John Bienenstock's group in Hamilton, looking at eosinophil colony forming cells, found cells which had basophils properties in what he termed eosinophil type colonies. In one series of experiments, he did it in such a way that the individual colonies were almost certainly clonal, and he still found this admixture, leading to the possibility that indeed there was a cell which could go either direction, i.e. to a basophil or an eosinophil. This would be quite in keeping with Ogawa's conception that development is a stochastic mechanism and that you can get almost any kind of a mixed colony in a given situation.

Spry: Jerry, can I have clarification. Did you say that you have a mast cell line that synthesizes MBP?

Gleich: Yes.

Spry: So, now we have to think of mast cells as a part of the MBP axis. Is this right?

Gleich: No. The mast cell line is from a patient with mast cell leukaemia. And with a tumour cell line one has to be very cautious. However, it happened at a time that we were writing a manuscript with Larry Lichtenstein on the observation that we did find MBP in basophils. We looked at mast cells also and did not see MBP. However, I recall very vividly at the time the proofs of that article arrived, we had the mast cell line expressing MBP, which gave us great pause, so we went back and looked at our original data again and felt that we were correct. We then proceeded to look at mast cells in a variety of situations and found that, if you took mast cells from normal skin, you did not see MBP in those mast cells. If you took mast cells from inflammatory areas or if you took mast cells from the gut, you did see MBP in them. We also saw variable MBP positivity in patients with urticaria pigmentosa. In some regions of the lesions the mast cells would be quite positive, in others they would be less positive. And this gradually led us to suspect that, in fact, this might not be synthesis, but rather akin to what Ann Dvorak has been talking about, i.e. endocytosis. We have now formally tested that by taking mast cells from lesions of the scalp, and incubating them in the presence of MBP, where the mast cells become positive. So, I think this represents the same phenomena that Ann Dvorak has studied, namely that the mast cell endocytoses the molecule.

Spry: So we can conclude that normally mast cells in man do not make MBP.

Sanderson: I'm going to take up this question of cell lineage that Jerry and Monique have mentioned. Obviously, if you go early enough, you'll find a cell that is pluripotential, as we know with IL-3. But from the work we've done with IL-5 and particularly the work from the Hall Institute using subclonal techniques, the eosinophil lineage is quite distinct from the basophil lineage and we never find basophils in liquid culture, where you've got a better chance of seeing different cell types. That's using single factor. But if you are using mixed factors, I'm not surprised that you get mixed colonies.

Gleich: I think the growth factor that Judah Denver used was a mononuclear cell supernatant and it undoubtedly is a real gemisch of all kinds of different things.

Sanderson: Even in these crude supernatants there are different factors that are involved in eosinophil and basophil lineage.

11

Eosinophils and Tissue Injury

C. J. F. Spry and P.-C. Tai

Department of Cellular and Molecular Sciences,
St. George's Hospital Medical School,
Cranmer Terrace, London SW17 0RE, UK

11.1 INTRODUCTION

Eosinophils are associated with a wide range of lesions in many different tissues (1). It is now thought that, in many of these disorders, eosinophils are responsible for inducing and/or maintaining reversible and irreversible changes in the areas of inflammation. This concept dates from experiments in the mid-1970s which showed that eosinophils are toxic for a number of parasites *in vitro* (2) and related experiments in which eosinophils were shown to be capable of degranulating (3) and damaging mammalian cells (4) and tissues *in vitro* (5).

Clinical work on patients who have large numbers of eosinophils in their blood and tissues, especially patients with the idiopathic hypereosinophilic syndrome (HES) (6), has shown that eosinophils often occur in association with thromboemboli, endomyocardial fibrosis (7), lymphatic diseases, gastro-

Eosinophils in Asthma
ISBN 0-12-506452-7

intestinal complications, coughing attacks and central and peripheral nervous system disease (8). Similar complications develop in patients with other diseases which produce an eosinophilia, such as tumour-associated eosinophilia (9), leukaemias and lymphomas, and hypersensitivity reactions. The presence of eosinophils in so many different settings suggest that they have a range of functions in human pathology.

Questions about the relative importance of eosinophils as either inhibitors of mast cell-mediated reactions (10), or pro-inflammatory cells, capable of damaging cells and tissues (3), are now largely resolved. It has been found that eosinophils have no unique mechanism for inhibiting mast cell responses (11). Indeed, it is clear that eosinophils can promote mast cell-, and basophil-mediated reactions (12), and are therefore best seen as a part of the effector limb of inflammatory responses.

The purpose of this review is to describe several types of tissue lesions which occur in association with a marked eosinophilia, and the deposition of eosinophil granule proteins, and to relate these to the properties, and effector functions of eosinophils as defined *in vitro*.

11.2   EOSINOPHILS AND RESPIRATORY DISEASES

Eosinophils are prominent in diseases affecting tissues with mucosal surfaces, especially the respiratory and gastrointestinal tracts. These are sites where inflammatory cells are believed to be important in protection against potentially pathogenic organisms. The discovery of eosinophils in the sputum of patients with asthma was made in about 1889 (13). This has become an area of considerable interest, with the demonstration of secreted eosinophil major basic protein (MBP), in the lungs (14) and sputum (15) of patients with asthma.

In the lungs, eosinophils are found around venules in the submucosa of the bronchi, with other inflammatory cells in interstitial lesions in granulomas (16) and in areas of focal damage. In asthma, eosinophils are submucosal, but may migrate into the bronchial lumen (17). Although eosinophils are usually seen in bronchoalveolar (BAL) washings from patients with asthma, they are present in smaller numbers than neutrophils, and the largest numbers of eosinophils are recovered in BAL from patients with eosinophilic pneumonia and fibrosing alveolitis. Histopathologists have long noted that eosinophils preferentially occupy the periphery of acute and chronic reactions in the lungs. We noted this in rats following the injection of parasites intravenously, when they lodged in pulmonary vessels, producing granulomas (18). However, it is now known that eosinophils can degranulate and so become difficult to identify by eosin staining. As a result, the number of eosinophils within granulomas may be underestimated, unless techniques are used to detect their secreted granule proteins such as eosinophil cationic protein (ECP), which can be deposited in large amounts in granulomas of the Churg–Strauss syndrome (19).

Respiratory symptoms occur in about 40% of patients with HES, and about 13% have lung infiltrates (6). They have coughing attacks, which are sometimes prominent at night and may be due to the sequestration of eosinophils within the vasculature of the lungs, as more eosinophils in venous blood than arterial blood have been found during the course of a coughing attack (Spry, C. J. 1982, unpublished observation). During these coughing attacks, the patients became breathless, but there was no alteration in FEV1, or in other respiratory function tests done at the bedside, showing that the syndrome was distinct from asthma.

Although allergic rhinitis, and asthma are the commonest causes of eosinophilia in western countries, they seldom precede the development of HES, and relatively few patients have been described with asthma and HES. The reasons for this are not clear. Most of the patients reported with lung involvement in HES have patchy infiltrates, often thought to be infectious in origin, but which resolve following treatment with steroids (20). They have been biopsied (21, 22), but show no specific features, and their pathogenesis is unknown. As patients with hypereosinophilia, and respiratory involvement seldom have classical asthma, the presence of eosinophils in the lung is not a sufficient condition for the induction of an asthmatic response.

A wide range of drug reactions can produce eosinophil infiltrates into the lungs without the development of asthma (23), although asthma is often seen in patients with cryptogenic pulmonary eosinophilia and granulomatous, and vasculitic diseases of the lungs. The relationship between eosinophils and these lung lesions remains to be discovered, but as Charcot–Leyden crystals are prominent within the lesions, and in the bronchi, it is probable that eosinophils are degranulating, and functioning as pro-inflammatory cells in these diseases.

11.3   EOSINOPHILS AND THROMBOEMBOLIC DISEASE

Thromboembolic complications are common in patients with hypereosinophilia. We noted this in our group of patients with HES (6), many of whom had retinal and choroidal lesions which were shown by fluorescent retinal angiography to be due to microvascular obstruction (24). Further studies demonstrated clotting defects in nine patients (25), which pointed to continuous, and usually subclinical, thrombotic events which occasionally led to large vessels occlusion.

Many patients with the HES have thrombi within their cardiac ventricular cavities (26), and these can sometimes embolize and produce major vessel occlusions. Splinter haemorrhages in the fingers and toes are common in these patients, and are believed to be produced by multiple small emboli from within the heart.

For these reasons, it is probable that one of the major toxic effects of eosinophils on tissues is via an effect on the coagulation system, as has been shown *in vitro* (27). This is not always inhibited by giving anti-coagulation, as several of our patients have developed major thrombi while taking warfarin.

11.4 EOSINOPHILS AND ENDOMYOCARDIAL FIBROSIS

The association between eosinophils and endomyocardial disease has been known for many years (28), but it was not until 1970 that it was suggested that eosinophils could be responsible for the tissue injury (29). Our work in this area has confirmed this, and we now feel that the presence of eosinophils and their granule products within the endomyocardium of patients with an eosinophilia of any cause, gives rise to myocardial damage and subsequent fibrosis (30). The initiating event for this process is still unknown. It has been suggested that thrombi may accumulate toxic eosinophil granule proteins at the endocardial surface. We have proposed that metabolic demands on the endomyocardium, which are different from the other parts of the heart may be linked in some way to the toxic effects of eosinophils in this site.

A recent study involving several groups has shown that eosinophil granule products, MBP, ECP and activated eosinophils were prominent within the heart in areas of myocardial damage, both in endomyocardial biopsies and in post-mortem samples from patients with endomyocardial disease (31). This adds to earlier information that degranulated eosinophils were present within the endomyocardium, as judged by electronmicroscopy, both in eosinophilic endomyocardial fibrosis, and the tropical form of the disease. The mechanisms which induce eosinophil secretion in these sites remain unknown.

11.5 EOSINOPHILS AND SKIN DISEASE

Eosinophils have a special place in the pathology of a wide range of skin disorders, ranging from pemphigus (32) to eczema. Eosinophils are also prominent in inflammatory lesions in the skin produced by parasites such as filaria and schistosomula. Eosinophils degranulate extensively within the skin in treated onchocerciasis, and atopic eczema (33). The amount of deposited eosinophil granule proteins seems out of proportion to the number of cells seen there histologically. The role of eosinophil constituents within the skin remains unknown. It has been reported that eosinophil MBP causes permeability changes when injected into normal human skin. However, an homogenate of eosinophil granules failed to produce a noticeable effect when injected into the skin of two of my patients.

There may be an association between eosinophils and Langerhans' cells in the skin. Eosinophils accumulated close to Langerhans' cells in the epidermis, following injection of environmental antigens in patients with atopic disease (35). The reasons for this association are not known, but it is possible that stimulated Langerhans' cells, may produce interleukin 1, which can induce GM-CSF production by vascular endothelial cells.

11.6 EOSINOPHILS AND VASCULAR PERMEABILITY

A relationship between eosinophils and episodic angioedema was first recorded in 1984 (34). A similar syndrome develops in patients injected with either recombinant IL-2 (36), or GM-CSF (37). They developed a marked eosinophilia and weight gain, both of which returned to normal when the injections were stopped. Two other diseases where eosinophils are associated with accumulations of fluid are the ascitic form of eosinophilic gastroenteritis (38), and certain types of pleural effusion association with marked increase in eosinophils (39).

11.7 EOSINOPHILS AND NEOPLASTIC DISEASE

The presence of large numbers of eosinophils in the blood and/or affected tissues in some patients with tumours has suggested that there may be a relationship between eosinophils and some malignant cells. These are: (1) endothelial cell tumours; (2) tumours involving Langerhans' cells (histiocytosis X); and (3) malignancies affecting T lymphocytes. It is possible that the occurrence of eosinophils in these diseases is related to the capacity of the neoplasms to produce molecules such as CSFs and cytokines, which affect the proliferation, localization and activation of eosinophils. These associations also raise the possibility that eosinophils may have a close relationship with these cell types in nonmalignant diseases. In the case of T cells, this relationship is well known. A link with endothelial cells has only been determined in the last few years (40), and it is probably due to their synthesis of GM-CSF which promotes several eosinophil functions (41). There is no work yet on possible relationships between eosinophils and Langerhans' cells, except that quoted above, and this may be an interesting area to explore in view of the common occurrence of eosinophils in patients with reticuloendotheliosis.

There are now several reports that the presence of eosinophils within tumours can be beneficial, but that a blood eosinophilia is a poor prognostic sign. This could be a reflection of the quantity of eosinopoietic factors produced within the tumour, or a toxic effect of eosinophils on the growth, or spread of tumour cells, but neither possibility has been tested experimentally.

The requirement for T cells in eosinopoiesis is now known to be linked to the capacity of lymphocytes to produce IL-5, which affects both eosinophil production and eosinophil activation. This may explain the association of eosinophils with many types of lymphomas. We recently reported an interesting association with lymphomatoid papulosis where there was hypereosinophilia and recurrent skin lesions, recurring over many years (33). In this disease the neoplastic T cells are clonal and the malignant process appears to be multifocal.

11.8   EOSINOPHIL INTERACTIONS WITH OTHER CELLS AND TISSUES

Although there have been reports on the capacity of eosinophils to damage cells *in vitro* (4), more work is needed to find the range of cells damaged by eosinophils *in vivo*. More is known about the range of stimuli which induce eosinophils to degranulate *in vitro*, and the activating factors which influence this. However, this has become a complex area, as it is now clear that two secretion signals are more effective than one, and that certain stimuli, especially those involving low-affinity receptors such as the IgE receptor, cause the secretion of only some of the granule constituents. It is possible that some granule constituents are more easily mobilized than others, so that relatively weak signals produce effects which are reversible; whereas a combination of a potent activating factor and secretagogue (such as complexed C3b) may induce the secretion of many molecules from eosinophils, which could have irreversible effects on adjacent cells, and tissues. Here again the final biological effect of inducing eosinophil secretion may be more complex than has been considered so far, as eosinophils may produce factors which affect neighbouring fibroblasts (43), accounting for the development of fibrosis in many chronic eosinophil-rich lesions.

11.9   MECHANISMS OF EOSINOPHIL-DEPENDENT TISSUE INJURY

The clinical evidence to incriminate eosinophils in the induction of tissue injury can be matched by an impressive list of individual eosinophil components, and their effects on cells and tissues. Each of the principal eosinophil granule constituents are now known to cause tissue damage (1), but the ways in which they do this are not known. The hypothesis that the highly basic proteins induce the formation of ion channels in cell membranes (44) is still open to question, as this has only been tested in liposomes.

11.10   CONCLUSION

It is concluded that studies on the complications which develop in patients with high blood eosinophil counts have brought to light several possible ways in which eosinophils may induce tissue lesions. Lymphocytes, endothelial cells, and possibly other interstitial cells appear to regulate their functions to a fine degree.

Clinical studies on patients with high eosinophil counts have shown that the presence of eosinophils alone is not sufficient to cause asthmatic reactions. However, once eosinophils have been induced to degranulate, they secrete a wide variety of effector molecules which give rise to a range of effects which may be reversible or permanent. In some clinical situations, eosinophils are probably present in tissues because of the inappropriate release of interleukins and other molecules which induce their proliferation and localization. Under these circumstances their effects on tissues may be deleterious. On the other hand, in allergic and inflammatory reactions due to potentially pathogenic organisms, eosinophils are likely to have a protective role. Unfortunately, there are many disorders in which the regulation of eosinophil production, and localization in tissue does not appear to confer significant benefits. These are clearly important areas for the development of new drugs, and new mechanisms for inhibiting the effect of eosinophils on cells and tissues.

Acknowledgements

We thank the Wellcome Trust, Medical Research Council, and British Heart Foundation for financial support, and our colleagues who have helped us to formulate some of the ideas put forward here.

REFERENCES

1. Spry, C. J. (1988). "Eosinophils. A Comprehensive Review and Guide to the Scientific and Medical Literature", 502. Oxford University Press, Oxford.
2. Butterworth, A. E. (1984). *Adv. Parasitol.* **23**, 143–235.
3. Spry, C. J. (1978). *Schweiz. Med. Wochenschr.* **108**, 1572–1576.
4. Gleich, G. J., Frigas, E., Loegering, D. A., Wassom, D. L. and Steinmuller, D. (1979). *J. Immunol.* **123**, 2925–2927.
5. Frigas, E., Loegering, D. A., Gleich, G. J. (1980). *Lab. Invest.* **42**, 35–43.
6. Spry, C. J. (1982). *Allergy* **37**, 539–551.
7. Spry, C. J. (1988). *In* "Immunological Aspects of Heart Diseases" (Ed. W. A. Littler), Clinical Immunology and Allergy 1.
8. Spry, C. J., Davies, J., Tai, P-C., Olsen, E.G., Oakley, C. M., Goodwin, J. F. (1983). *Q. J. Med.* **52**, 1–22.
9. Lowe, D., Jorio, J. and Hutt, M. S. (1981). *J. Clin. Pathol.* **34**, 1343–1348.
10. Austen, K. F. (1978). *J. Immunol.* **121**, 793–805.
11. Weller, P. F., Wasserman, S. I., Austen, K. F. (1980). *In* "The Eosinophil in Health and Disease" (Eds A. A. Mahmoud, K. F. Austen and A. S. Simon), 115–130. Grune and Stratton, New York.
12. O'Donnell, M. C., Ackerman, S. J., Gleich, G. J., Thomas, L. L. (1983). *J. Exp. Med.* **157**, 1981–91.
13. Gollasch, Dr. (1889). *Fortschritte der Medizin* (Berlin) **7**, 361–365.
14. Filley, W. V., Holley, K. E., Kephart, G. M., Gleich, G. J. (1982). *Lancet* **2**, 11–6.
15. Gleich, G. J. (1986). *Bull. Eur. Physiopathol. Respir.* **22** (Suppl. 7), 62–69.
16. Lanham, J. G., Elkon, K. B., Pusey, C. D., Hughes, G. R. (1984). *Medicine* (Baltimore) **63**, 65–81.
17. Gleich, G. J., Motojima, S., Frigas, E., Kephart, G. M., Fujisawa, T. and Kravis, L. P. (1987). *J. Allergy Clin. Immunol.* **80**, 412–415.
18. Boyer, M. H., Spry, C. J., Beeson, P. B. and Sheldon, W. H. (1971). *Yale J. Biol. Med.* **43**, 351–357.
19. Tai, P.-C., Holt, M. E., Denny, P., Gibbs, A. R., Williams, B. D. and Spry, C. J. (1984). *Br. Med. J. (Clin. Res.)* **289**, 400–402.
20. Epstein, D. M., Taormina, V., Gefter, W. B., Miller, W. T. (1981). *Radiology* **140**, 59–62.

21. Hill, R., Wang, N. S. and Berry, G. (1984). *Angiology* **35**, 238–244.
22. Edwards, D., Wald, J. A., Dobozin, B. S. and Kirkpatrick, C. H. (1987). *N. Engl. J. Med.* **317**, 573–574.
23. Spry, C. J. (1980). *Clin. Haematol.* **9**, 521–534.
24. Chaine, G., Davies, J., Kohner, E. M., Hawarth, S. and Spry, C. J. (1982). *Ophthalmology* **89**, 1348–1356.
25. Davies, J., Powell, D., McCall, E., Hegde, G. and Spry, C. J. (1989). (Submitted)
26. Davies, J., Spry, C. J., Sapsford, R., Olsen, E. G., de Perez, G., Oakley, C. M. and Goodwin, J. F. (1983). *O. J. Med.* **52**, 23–39.
27. Venge, P., Dahl, R. and Hallgren, R. (1979). *Thromb. Res.* **14**, 641–649.
28. Löffler, W. (1936). *Schweiz. Med. Wochenschr.* **17**, 817–820.
29. Brockington, I. F., Luzzatto, L. and Osunkoya, B. O. (1970). *Afr. J. Med. Sci.* **1**, 343–352.
30. Spry, C. J. (1987). *In* "Pathogenesis of myocarditis and cardiomyopathy: recent experimental and clinical studies" (Eds C. Kawai and W. A. Abelmann), 293–310. Cardiomyopathy Update 1. University of Tokyo Press, Tokyo.
31. Tai, P.-C., Ackerman, S. J., Spry, C. J., Dunnette, S., Olsen, E. G. and Gleich, G. J. (1987) *Lancet* **1**, 643–647.
32. Razzaque Ahmed A. (1984). *J. Cutan. Pathol.* **11**, 237–248.
33. Whittaker, S. J., Jones, R. R. and Spry, C. J. (1988). *J. Am. Acad. Dermatol.* **18**, 339–344.
35. Gleich, G. J., Schroeter, A. L., Marcoux, J. P., Sachs, M. I., O'Connell, E. J. and Kohler, P. F. (1984). *N. Engl. J. Med.* **310**, 1621–1626.
36. Bruynzeel Kooman, C., van Wichen, D. F., Spry, C. J., Venge, P. and Bruynzeel, P. (1987). *Br. J. Dermatol.* (in press)
37. Kern, P. and Deitrich, M. (1986). *Blut.* **52**, 249–254.
38. Groopman, J. E., Mitsuyasu, R. T., DeLeo, M.J., Oette, D.H. and Golde, D.W. (1987). *N. Engl. J. Med.* **317**, 593–598.
39. Spry, C. J. (1984). *In* "Textbook of Gastroenterology" (Eds I. A. Bouchier, R. N. Hodgson and M. R. Keighley), 596–598. Baillière Tindall, London.
40. Martensson, G., Pettersson, K. and Thiringer, G. (1985). *Eur. J. Respir. Dis.* **67**, 326–334.
41. Rothenberg, M. E., Owen, W. F. Jr., Silberstein, D. S., Soberman, R. J., Austen, K. F. and Stevens, R. L. (1987). *Science* **237**, 645–647.
42. Begley, C. G., Lopez, A. F., Nicola, N. A., Warren, D. J., Vadas, M. A., Sanderson, C. J. and Metcalf, D. (1986). *Blood* **68**, 162–166.
43. Pincus, S. H., Ramesh, K. S. and Wyler, D. J. (1987). *Blood* **70**, 572–574.
44. Young, J. D., Petersson, C. G., Venge, P. and Cohn, Z. A. (1986). *Nature* **321**, 613–616.

DISCUSSION

Vargaftig (Chairman)

Gleich: I'm particularly intrigued by your association, which I hadn't thought about, I must confess, between the formation of oedema in the ascites form of eosinophilic gastroenteritis and the cutaneous situation, because they are parallels it seems to me. Now, you didn't touch upon this, but there is another parallel, Patients who, in the States we have this great excitement about treating patients with malignant disease using IL-2, develop florid eosinophilia; and in at least one of those cases we've seen an histologic picture by immunofluorescence of MBP deposition in tissues. I wanted to ask you about the existence of the small granules, which Spicer and his colleague described. As I remember their studies, they showed acid phosphatase and aryl sulphatase in those granules. There were some earlier studies out of Polote's laboratory that showed acid phosphatase in the crystalloid-containing granules, but it appeared to be in a latent form. You had to do something to the eosinophil to reveal it, so that when you came down to the difference between the crystalloid-containing granules and the small granules of Spicer, one is left with the aryl sulphatase. But, I didn't quite get the point. Why do you query their distinction?

Spry: The reason I am making a little bit of a meal of this, is that Per Venge would like us to think that there are different types of granules in the eosinophil based on the isopicnic gradient separation of disrupted eosinophils. This is a very tempting line to take. The immunocytochemical and histochemical data show that the small granules have ECP in them; they also have peroxidase aryl sulphatase and acid phosphatase in an active enzymatic form. The large granule does not have enzymatic acid phosphatase; although the enzyme is present, it's just not fully functional. I don't think it can work under the hypotonic conditions present in the matrix. There is of course peroxidase there, which again doesn't stain quite so well as in the small granule where it is enzymatically even more active. So the differences between these two granules are their size and their content of aryl sulphatase. Per: if you plot the peroxidase concentration in your slide with a bigger ordinate, do you find bumps of peroxidase corresponding to those ECP peaks that you showed us? Is there no peroxidase in those extra little peaks?

Venge: No, actually not, but I would also like to comment. I don't totally disagree, I think it's very likely that we may have one major granule population and that the other forms we see are derived from this major one. This may actually have a bearing on the differential secretion of these proteins. In some situations you may have packaging of the proteins in secretory granules lacking peroxidase. In other situations maybe there is peroxidase included as well. In some patients we have only seen one compartment with peroxidase and we have seen the three additional compartments separated on density gradients with ECP and EPX.

Spry: Right.

Sanjar: This is a question about all forms of eosinophils—normodense and hypodense. Is there any evidence to suggest that eosinophils are produced or not produced in the hypodense form to start with rather than be normodense and then be transformed?

Spry: I was hoping that somebody would have answered that question who is actually using those density gradients on bone marrow. I think Dr Fukuda is the only one who has fractionated marrow with Percoll gradients and found light density cells. Were these immature cells or mature cells. Perhaps Dr Fukuda could answer that.

Fukuda: Immature cells from bone marrow show hypodensity.

Sanderson: Yes, I want to respond to that because as Matthew pointed out before, this question of density is a very complicated thing. One of the main causes of changes of density in cells is the nuclear cytoplasmic ratio. Now, that might not be the reason for the production of hypodense mature eosinophils, but I think the immature cells in the bone marrow which are blastoform cells with a very large nucleus are quite different in structure to the mature eosinophil. You could well have hypodense cells in bone marrow in the terms that you are measuring them, but it might have nothing to do with the hypodense cells you are seeing in the tissue and blood. I think they are quite different situations.

Kay: I enjoyed your talk very much and certainly agree with you that the tissue damage in association with the eosinophils is variable, but I got slightly worried at the beginning of your talk that you were making inferences about tissue damage from your findings in the hypereosinophilic syndrome. I want to emphasize that you can not in my opinion draw any conclusions about the nature of tissue injury in one disease from findings in another. There are lots of paradoxes about asthma. We have to explain why it is that in many forms of the disease there is substantial infiltration of eosinophils in and around the bronchial epithelium, and free eosinophils in the lumen, yet the disease is extremely mild. You can find quite severe inflammatory changes in the presence of very mild disease. In allergic bronchopulmonary aspergillosis there is proximal bronchiectasis with florid eosinophilic infiltration in bronchi and acini. Then in idiopathic pulmonary eosinophilia or cryptogenic pulmonary eosinophilia there is massive stuffing of the alveoli with the eosinophils and yet, following treatment, absolutely remarkably normal looking parenchymal lung tissue. As well as the fantastically complex interactions between the bone marrow turnover of these cells, the messages which are coming from tissue sites, the nature of these signals, what the actual micro-environment does to the cells and what they secrete, I'm always faced with the problem that inflammation is a repair process as well.

Spry: I agree entirely. In bronchoalveolar lavage studies done in Japan, the highest number of eosinophils in bronchoalveolar lavage come from patients with eosinophilic pneumonia. Second in the league table are patients who've got aspirin sensitivity and classic asthma of the kind we've been discussing today is near the bottom of the league table. On the repair mechanisms there have been some suggestions by Dr Bassett in New Zealand about this and her studies over the years have not been very convincing for me, although others may disagree.

Wasserman: A comment on literature reviews and then a question. What gets into the literature is what people think is interesting and unusual, so that you don't see as many papers on, say, the association of IgE and eosinophilia, which we assume exists, as on the dichotomy between those two. We have to watch for the bias in the literature and for the bias of the reviewer. That's just an aside.

The issue on different granules in the eosinophil is of some interest. We certainly know that there are at least three different granules in the human neutrophil which are clearly different by their constituents, by their pattern, by their isolation. The eosinophil granule is, as you point out, very much more interesting and it is difficult to differentiate whether these granules are, as Per Venge suggests and as you suggest, different granules and/or granules modified during their lifespan. The proteins are made in the golgi and then packaged into the granules; alternating secretion due to factors which we do not yet understand could lead to granules with a different history. The second possibility is that the granule once packaged can be secondarily modified, thus leading to generation of new granules. Is there any evidence on those points?

Spry: Well, as far as I know, nobody has done any biosynthetic studies comparing HES and leukaemic eosinophils and normal bone marrow eosinophils for their capacity to make different amounts of these different proteins. I think if you wanted to postulate that there could be differential control of protein synthesis, you might find under those three conditions that some bone marrows made a lot of ECP, some made a lot of MBP and others did other things.

Wasserman: And I am suggesting that eosinophils might at different periods in its own lifespan make all three in equal amounts and then, for one reason or another, suppress or activate its ability to make a different protein so that you would see different ratios and different granules based on what input the cell was receiving.

Spry: There is very, very little mRNA in the fully granulated eosinophil. There is a little bit for repair proteins presumably.

Wasserman: No, no, exactly, so that as the eosinophil is being produced, what you're seeing in the differential granulation is the history of the eosinophil when it was a synthetic cell. The other comment I wanted to make was with regard to tissue injury and eosinophil accumulation. You can see eosinophils and no injury and you can see injury with eosinophils. It suggests that there are differential stimuli for accumulation and activation, and some stimuli are sufficient both to accumulate and to activate the eosinophils, and other stimuli are sufficient to accumulate but not cause grave degrees of activation, and that you need both to get the kinds of inflammatory changes that cause tissue injury.

Spry: Well, I've been struck by the fact that there are few stimuli which don't cause secretion.

Wasserman: Well, but maybe the amount of secretion and again the pattern of secretion can vary. It's like the problem we have with the mast cell, where people assume that if you can find histamine, the mast cell has been activated, but when you talk about 20 or 25 mediators being potentially generated by a single cell, looking at one may be very misleading.

Spry: Yes, yes, I'm sure that's right.

Dahl: A comment about the presence of eosinophils in tissues and damage. We have some indirect evidence from histological processing of tissues, looking for granules and their secretory products, that eosinophils can be present in tissues without secreting, but if secretion does occur there is always damage.

You commented that asthmatics cannot have hypereosinophilic syndrome. From my practice I have seen patients who presented with asthma for some years, and then developed the hypereosinophilic syndrome but, of course, then they are not asthmatics any more. You find that 40% of patients with HES have lung symptoms, do you know if all patients with the hypereosinophilic syndrome have eosinophils in their lungs or is it only those who have lung symptoms, and do you know what their histamine reactivity is?

Spry: No, we've done a large panel of respiratory function tests on our patients with HES, because some years back Barry Kay was very interested in this issue of asthma in hypereosinophilic patients. We found very little evidence for reversible bronchoconstriction in any of the twelve we studied. There has been little work as far as I know on the histology of the lung in patients with the hypereosinophilic syndrome or bronchoalveolar lavage in this condition, except when they've had eosinophilic pneumonia when, naturally, eosinophils were found.

12

Pharmacological Modulation of Eosinophil Accumulation in Guinea-pig Airways

S. Sanjar, I. Colditz, S. Aoki, K. Boubekeur and J. Morley

Preclinical Research,
Sandoz AG,
CH 4002 Basel, Switzerland

12.1 INTRODUCTION

An infiltrate of eosinophils in the bronchial walls and airways of subjects dying from asthma was recognized over 60 years ago. Even though the evidence from histopathology was unequivocal, eosinophils attracted little attention and their role in asthma pathogenesis was demoted in consequence of the recognition that histamine, a powerful spasmogen of airway smooth muscle, was released when mast cells were activated by agents such as allergen (1). Interest in the eosinophil was revived in the 1970s following description of eosinophil chemotactic factor of anaphylaxis (ECF-A) as a product released from sensitized lungs during an acute allergic reaction (2).

Eosinophils in Asthma
ISBN 0-12-506452-7

The chemotactic activity of ECF-A has been attributed to tetrapeptides valine– and alanine–glycine–serine–glutamine (3). These peptides have chemotactic activity for eosinophils, but such chemotactic activity is unimpressive when compared with C5a, platelet activating factor (PAF) or leukotriene B_4 (4, 5, 6, 7). Activation and tissue localization of eosinophils is also evident in some responses of cellular immunity, and crude lymphokine preparations with chemotactic activity for eosinophils have been identified (8, 9, 10, 11). The molecules responsible for the activity have not been purified to homogeneity and cloned. However, if the potency of these lymphokines is comparable to other biological activities of lymphokines, it may be expected that these substances will prove to be the most potent endogenous stimulants of eosinophil migration. At present, the mediators of eosinophil infiltration of bronchial tissues in asthmatics remain unknown.

Despite an association between eosinophils and asthma, drugs have not been selected on the basis of their capacity to inhibit accumulation of eosinophils. Dominance of the mast cell in theories of asthma pathogenesis has contributed largely to this situation, especially as such ideas included the notion that eosinophils played a beneficial role in immediate hypersensitivity reactions by inactivating mediators such as histamine and peptidoleukotrienes (12). A further limitation to the selection of drugs to inhibit eosinophil accumulation in asthmatic lungs and in other inflammatory conditions has been the absence of an adequate model to describe the mechanism by which eosinophils are stimulated to enter inflammatory lesions.

12.2   A MODEL OF GRANULOCYTE MIGRATION INTO ACUTE INFLAMMATORY LESIONS

From the earliest studies of acute inflammation it was acknowledged that chemotaxis of leucocytes may contribute to their accumulation in inflammatory lesions (13). Chemotaxis of leucocytes is a functional definition of locomotor behaviour of cells *in vitro* (14). The notion that chemotaxis may be the major determinant of granulocyte emigration from blood vessels into sites of inflammation *in vivo* has been undermined by the observation that inflammatory lesions become desensitized to chemotactic agents with a high degree of stimulus specificity (15, 16, 17) and by recent advances in the understanding of adhesion events between granulocytes and inflamed endothelium (18, 19). Current studies indicate that there are two patterns of granulocyte adhesion to endothelium during inflammatory reactions *in vivo*: immediate adhesion that occurs within minutes of application of chemotactic agents such as LTB_4,

PAF, C5a and f-Met-Leu-Phe; and delayed adhesion that commences around 30 min after application of agents such as interleukin-1, endotoxin and casein (20). *In vivo* studies have recently shown that local treatment with inhibitors of protein synthesis prevent the latter, but not the former, pattern of interaction between granulocyte and endothelium (21). From such studies, a model has emerged which identifies three critical events in neutrophil emigration:

1. initial adhesion of intravascular neutrophils to endothelium that has been induced to express adhesive domains by extravascular inflammatory agents;
2. possible locomotor activation of neutrophils by the adhesive event leading to emigration between endothelial cells; then
3. extravascular tissue localization of neutrophils, directed in part by chemotactic agents, and under the constraints imposed by tissue architecture (22).

An important component of this model is the concept that emigration of neutrophils is initiated by local production of pro-inflammatory mediators in the tissue rather than within the vascular compartment. Eosinophils share many characteristics with neutrophils, including similar chemotactic responses to PAF, LTB$_4$ and C5a (5). A preliminary study indicates that these cells also bind avidly to activated endothelial cells *in vitro* by the same molecular determinants as neutrophils (23). Thus, the current model of neutrophil emigration provides a starting point for investigating the mechanism for tissue localization of eosinophils.

12.3   PAF-INDUCED EOSINOPHIL ACCUMULATION IN BRONCHIAL AIRWAYS

Studies on the inflammatory potential of PAF *in vivo* have shown that it induces increased vascular permeability and infiltration of leucocytes when injected intracutaneously (24), and platelet and leucocyte aggregation when injected intravenously (25). Experimental evidence accumulated over the last eight years has also shown that exposure of animals or humans to PAF can reproduce many of the clinical findings of asthma (26). Following intratracheal instillation of PAF in baboons, there is a selective accumulation of eosinophils in the lumen of bronchial airways (27). The capacity of ketotifen, but not pyribenzamine, to inhibit such eosinophil accumulation (27) led us to develop an assay of PAF-induced eosinophil accumulation in bronchial airways of the guinea-pig. We have used this system to investigate the capacity of classical anti-asthma drugs to inhibit eosinophil accumulation.

Guinea-pigs were housed in 4-litre plexiglass chambers and exposed to an

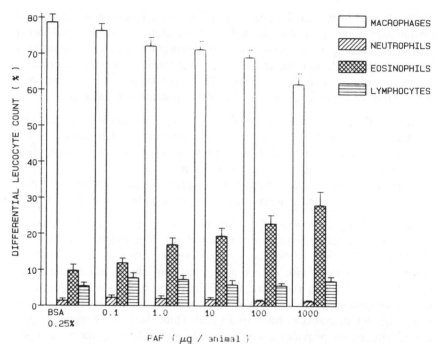

Fig. 1   Differential leucocyte counts in bronchoalveolar lavage fluid 48 hours after exposure of guinea-pigs to aerosols of platelet activating factor (PAF) or bovine serum albumen (PAF carrier). The total leucocyte count in bronchoalveolar lavage fluid of control animals was $20.8 \pm 2.4 \times 10^6$ cells/ml ($n = 10$). No significant change in total leucocyte count occurred in treatment animals (10 animals per treatment group).

aerosol of PAF generated by a Devilbiss nebulizer for 1 h with an air flow of 7 1/min. To assess the cellular inflammatory response in the airways, animals were killed by an intraperitoneal injection of barbiturate, the trachea was cannulated and six serial infusions of Ca^{2+}-free and Mg^{2+}-free Tyrode containing EDTA and 0.25% bovine serum albumen were used to wash inflammatory cells from the airway lumen. Total cell counts were made with a haemocytometer and differential cell counts were made on cell smears stained with Leishman's stain. A selective, dose-dependent eosinophil accumulation was observed 48 h after exposure to between 1 μg and 1 mg of PAF (28; Fig. 1).

Although the concentrations of PAF may appear to be high, it is predicted that approximately 0.01% of the aerosol dose enters the airways of guinea-pigs (29). No increase in the number of neutrophils was observed and the only other change was a decline in macrophage numbers as eosinophil numbers increased. Total cell numbers did not increase following exposure to PAF. Depletion of platelets or neutrophils by intravenous injection of specific antisera had no effect on eosinophil accumulation. The kinetics of the eosinophil influx were examined and a biphasic pattern was observed. Maximal eosinophil numbers were recovered 48 h after exposure to PAF. The eosinophil numbers in bronchoalveolar lavage fluid (BAL) subsequently declined, returning to baseline level between 1 and 2 weeks. Intense eosinophil accumulation occurred in the first 4 h after PAF exposure and accounted for 49% of the total number of eosinophils recovered in BAL at 48 h. A second peak of eosinophil accumulation was observed between 24 and 48 h, when a further 46% of the eosinophils recovered at 48 hours entered the airways accessible by bronchoalveolar lavage.

12.4   BRONCHIAL EOSINOPHILIA FOLLOWING PARENTERAL INJECTION OF PAF

The effect of intraperitoneal or subcutaneous injection of PAF was also examined in guinea-pigs. The intracutaneous route resulted in local accumulation of leucocytes amongst which neutrophils predominated. Following intraperitoneal injection of PAF, there was initially infiltration of the peritoneal cavity by neutrophils. Eosinophils appeared later in the inflammatory exudate and outnumbered neutrophils after 24 h. Both routes of administration resulted in the accumulation of eosinophils in bronchial airways but, as with PAF inhalation, no increase in neutrophils was evident in BAL. Greatest numbers of eosinophils were recovered in bronchoalveolar washes 24 h after administration of PAF intraperitoneally. The finding that subcutaneous or intraperitoneal injection of PAF induced an accumulation of eosinophils in the lungs of guinea-pigs provides a further discrepancy with the hypothesis that chemotactic mechanisms account for such tissue localization of eosinophils. In this instance, it seems highly improbable that there is a positive chemotactic gradient of PAF from the vessel wall into the extravascular tissue spaces of the lungs. Furthermore, these findings are in discord with the observation that neutrophil emigration is initiated by pro-inflammatory mediators generated locally within the inflamed tissue (*vide supra*). Thus, an alternative explanation must be envisaged in order to account for selective eosinophil accumulation in bronchial airways, and it may be presumed that the capacity of eosinophils to emigrate from blood vessels can be determined by mediators which affect eosinophils within the systemic circulation.

   In addition to our observations using PAF, there are three pieces of evidence which support this proposition. Eosinophils, like neutrophils, are distributed within the vascular compartment in marginating and circulating pools (30). Eosinophils in the two pools are in dynamic equilibrium and the intravascular half-life of these cells is of the order of 12 h (12, 30). It is known that injection of cortisol induces a marked eosinopenia which lasts several hours and is presumed to be due to movement of eosinophils into the marginal pool. However, Sabag *et al.* (31) observed infiltration by eosinophils of the spleen and the tissue matrix of lymph nodes and thymus, but not other tissues, following injection of cortisol in rats. Thus, injection of cortisol induced eosinophils to leave the circulating and marginating pools and to accumulate selectively within certain lymphoid tissues. There is also intense infiltration of the endometrium during the oestrogen-dominant phase of the oestrous cycle in rodents (32). This migratory response of eosinophils can be induced in ovarectomized rats by oestrogen, and Tchernitchin and Galand found that eosinophil accumulation correlated with oestrogen concentrations in blood but not in endometrial tissue (32). Finally, Bass *et al.* (33) observed that intravenous injection of C5a and f-Met-Leu-Phe in rabbits caused a transient neutropenia lasting 10–30 min, whereas eosinopenia was still evident 5 h after treatment. The eosinopenia could not be accounted for by release of endogenous cortisol. These three events may reflect eosinophil emigration from blood vessels following intravascular activation of the cells, though the possibility that eosinophil emigration is a consequence of local production of eosinophil chemotactic factors in distant tissues following systemic permeation of the PAF, cortisol, oestrogen or chemotactic factors has not been formally excluded by these studies.

Our findings of bronchial eosinophilia following parenteral injection of PAF concur with a recent histological study of the cellular changes in the airways of guinea pigs following intravenous injection of PAF in which Lellouch-Tubiana *et al.* (34) observed pronounced eosinophil accumulation in the bronchial walls but not in alveoli. This observation mimics one of the important histological findings in bronchial asthma. It should be noted that the blood supply to the bronchi comes from the left heart whereas the granulocyte aggregation that follows intravenous PAF injection occurs in the pulmonary capillaries fed by the right heart (25). Thus, following intravenous injection of PAF, eosinophils, after first aggregating in the alveolar vasculature (25), must disaggregate, pass through the left heart and then emigrate when they are within bronchial venules. The molecular basis for this high degree of site-specificity for eosinophil emigration has not been investigated. A central role for PAF as the final mediator of bronchial eosinophil extravasation seems unlikely in view of the failure of PAF to induce marked eosinophil emigration when injected intradermally in normal subjects (24). Furthermore, PAF is produced readily by endothelial cells *in vitro* following stimulation by diverse agents including thrombin, bradykinin, histamine,

Table 1   Effect of anti-asthma drugs on the accumulation of eosinophils in guinea-pig airways 48 h after exposure to PAF by aerosol

Drug	Dose[a] (mg/kg/day)	Inhibition of response[b] (%)	Probability[c]
Ketotifen	1.0	50.0 ± 4.5	<0.001
	0.1	36.9 ± 4.0	<0.001
Aminophylline	10.0	53.6 ± 9.0	<0.001
Disodium cromoglicate	1.0	39.6 ± 9.0	<0.01
Dexamethasone	1.0	60.4 ± 4.5	<0.001
Azelastine	1.0	28.4 ± 9.0	<0.01
Mepyramine	2.0	8.1 ± 13.5	n.s.
Indomethacin	1.0	15.3 ± 4.5	n.s.
Salbutamol	1.0	13.5 ± 9.0	n.s.
AH 21-132	1.0	55.9 ± 3.6	<0.001
	0.1	20.3 ± 4.5	<0.05

[a] Drugs were administered for 5 days by subcutaneous implant before animals were exposed to an aerosol of PAF (100 μg). Eosinophil responses were assessed 2 days later by bronchoalveolar lavage.
[b] Eosinophils (4.35 ± 0.49 × 10^7 cells) in bronchoalveolar lavage fluid from animals receiving saline implants constituted 22.2 ± 2.0% of the harvested cells.
[c] Probability v. control by student's t test.

leukotrienes and interleukin 1 (35), despite the failure of these agents to induce selective, or in some cases any, eosinophil accumulation in inflammatory lesions *in vivo*. Clearly the mechanisms underlying the pulmonary localization of eosinophils are largely unknown and the role of inflammatory mediators in this phenomenon requires further clarification.

12.5 EFFECT OF ANTI-ASTHMA DRUGS ON PAF-INDUCED BRONCHIAL EOSINOPHILIA

In order to examine the capacity of anti-asthma drugs to modify eosinophil accumulation in the bronchial airways, guinea-pigs received a subcutaneous implant of drugs in sustained release, miniosmotic pumps (Alzet) over a 7 day period. After 5 days, animals were exposed to an aerosol of PAF (100 μg) and inflammatory exudates were collected 2 days later by bronchoalveolar lavage. The inhibition of PAF-induced eosinophilia by anti-asthma drugs is presented in Table 1. Ketotifen caused significant inhibition at doses of 0.1 mg/kg/d and 1.0 mg/kg/d. Other drugs which inhibited eosinophil influx to a significant extent were aminophylline, disodium cromoglicate, dexamethasone, azelastine and AH21-132; whereas mepyramine, indomethacin and salbutamol proved ineffective.

The present results imply that an important component of the prophylactic activity in asthma of established prophylactic anti-asthma drugs may be an ability to inhibit bronchial eosinophilia. This property of aminophylline, cromoglicate, dexamethasone and ketotifen is additional to the ability of these drugs to inhibit the development of the bronchial hyperreactivity that accompanies exposure to PAF (36). The capacity of drugs to inhibit eosinophil accumulation and airway hyperreactivity may be predictive of prophylactic efficacy in asthma. AH21-132 is a novel anti-asthma drug which shares these properties in preclinical studies (37, 38) and hence will test the validity of the association revealed by the present study on eosinophils and the earlier studies on airway reactivity.

12.6   MECHANISMS OF INHIBITION OF BRONCHIAL EOSINOPHILIA

The mechanisms by which drugs inhibit the accumulation of eosinophils in bronchial airways is unclear. At least four modes of action can be envisaged.

First, the number of eosinophils available to enter inflammatory lesions may be limited due to suppression of eosinophilopoiesis. Production of eosinophils by bone marrow appears to be driven by two mechanisms; a basal, non-immunological pathway (12) and a T cell dependent pathway that leads to amplified and accelerated maturation of eosinophils (39, 40). *In vitro*, it has been reported that corticosteroids can suppress the maturation of eosinophils from pluripotential stem cells through an action on T cells, which results in elevated numbers of neutrophil colonies and decreased numbers of eosinophil colonies (41, 42). However, the suppressive effect of hydrocortisone on eosinophilopoiesis was found to be independent of an action on accessory cells in a second study, so that this issue remains unresolved (43).

Secondly, drugs may inhibit the capacity of eosinophils to adhere to a substratum. Active adhesion to endothelium is an important step in the emigration of leucocytes as evidenced by failure of granulocytes to extravasate in patients with genetic deficiency of the granulocyte adhesive glycoprotein p150,95. *In vitro*, corticosteroids inhibit the adhesion of eosinophils to substrata (44). This observation may conflict with evidence of eosinopenia due to steroid exposure, which involves passive adhesion to endothelium during margination, and perhaps also active adhesion and emigration as discussed above.

Thirdly, drugs may inhibit the locomotor capacity of eosinophils. Cytostatic and cytotoxic drugs, phenothiazines and a number of antibiotics have this activity (44), in addition to corticosteroids, although the concentrations of steroids reported in the literature exceed therapeutic doses (44). Disodium cromoglicate suppresses the up-regulation of complement and IgG (Fc) receptors that is observed when neutrophils, eosinophils and monocytes are treated with the chemotactic peptide, f-Met-Leu-Phe (45). Receptor up-regulation, an integral component of the chemotactic response of leucocytes, is inhibited by disodium cromoglicate which may contribute to the capacity of disodium cromoglicate to inhibit eosinophil chemotaxis *in vitro* (A. B. Kay, this meeting) and to retard eosinophil influx into the lung as evidenced by a suppression of eosinophil numbers in the sputum of asthmatics (46).

Finally, drugs may inhibit the generation of extracellular mediators involved in the evolution of an eosinophilic inflammatory response. Again, corticosteroids exhibit this property by suppressing the release of monokines and lymphokines from stimulated mononuclear leucocytes (47) and by suppressing production of PAF (48). In a recent study, ketotifen, at doses of 1 μg/ml and greater, suppressed PAF production by human neutrophils, whereas disodium cromoglicate and tranilast were inactive (49).

A further effect of drugs on eosinophils that may be of relevance to therapy of asthma is their ability to inhibit activation of eosinophils and the release of granular contents. Preventing the accumulation of eosinophils in bronchial airways, however, should circumvent the need for "stabilizing" eosinophils. The present model of PAF-induced eosinophil accumulation in guinea-pig airways should facilitate studies of the factors regulating the migration of eosinophils and the pharmacological regulation of this component of the asthma response.

12.7   CONCLUSION

We have demonstrated that exposure to PAF by aerosol or by parenteral injection induces a selective accumulation of eosinophils in airways of guinea-pigs and thus reproduces an important element of clinical asthma. The ability of parenteral (subcutaneous and intraperitoneal) injections of PAF to induce migration of eosinophils into airways is discordant with the current model of regulation of granulocyte migration into inflammatory lesions by mediators generated locally within the site of inflammation. This finding implies that PAF may act systemically on eosinophils to modify their migratory destiny. The classical prophylactic anti-asthma drugs inhibited PAF-induced eosinophil accumulation, whereas symptomatic anti-asthma drugs and other drug categories were found to be without such action. It therefore is likely that the ability of drugs to inhibit eosinophil accumulation in bronchial airways is an important component of prophylactic protection against asthma.

REFERENCES

1. Riley, J. F. and West, G. B. (1963). The occurrence of histamine in mast cells. *In* "Handbook of Experimental Pharmacology" (Eds O. Eichler and A. Farah), 431–481. Springer, Berlin.
2. Kay, A. B. and Austen, K. F. (1971). The IgE-mediated release of an eosinophil leucocyte chemotactic factor from human lung. *J. of Immunol.* **197**, 899–902.
3. Goetzl, E. J. and Austen, K. F. (1976). Structural determinants of the eosinophil chemotactic activity of the acidic tetrapeptides of eosinophil chemotactic factor of anaphylaxis. *J. of Exp. Med.* **144**, 1424–1437.
4. Wardlaw, A. J., Moqbel, R., Cromwell, O. and Kay, A. B. (1986). Platelet-Activating Factor. A potent chemotactic and chemokinetic factor for human eosinophils. *J. of Clin. Invest.* **78**, 1701–1706.
5. Hakansson, L., Westerlund, D. and Venge, P. (1987). New method for the measurement of eosinophil migration. *J. Leukocyte Biol.* **42**, 689–696.
6. Tamura, N., Argawal, D. K., Suliaman, F. A. and Townley, R. G. (1987). Effects of platelet activating factor on the chemotaxis of normodense eosinophils from normal subjects. *Biochem. Biophys. Res. Comm.* **142**, 638–644.
7. Czarnetzki, B. M. and Rosenbach, T. (1986). Chemotaxis of human neutrophils and eosinophils towards leukotriene B_4 and its 20-w-oxidation products *in vitro*. *Prostaglandins* **31**, 851–858.
8. Cohen, S. and Ward P. A. (1971). Experimental eosinophilia III. *In vitro* and *in vivo* activity of a lymphocyte and immune complex-dependent chemotactic factor for eosinophils. *J. Exp. Med.* **133**, 133–146.
9. Colley, D. C. (1973). Eosinophils and immune mechanisms I. Eosinophil stimulation factor (ESP): a lymphokine induced by specific antigen or phytohaemagglutinin. *J. Immunol.* **110**, 1419–1429.
10. Torisu, M., Yoshida, T. and Ward, P. A. (1973). Lymphocyte derived eosinophil chemotactic factor. II. Studies on the mechanism of activation of the precursor substances by immune complexes. *J. Immunol.* **111**, 1450–1458.
11. Colley, D. C. (1976). Eosinophils and immune mechanisms IV. Culture conditions, antigen requirements, production kinetics and immunologic specificity of the lymphokine eosinophil stimulation promoter. *Cell. Immunol.* **24**, 328–339.
12. Weller, P. F. and Goetzl, E. J. (1979). The regulatory and effector roles of eosinophils. *Adv. in Immunol.* **27**, 339–371.
13. Metchnikoff, E. (1893). "Lectures on the Comparative Pathology of Inflammation". Kegan Paul, Trench, Trubner, London.
14. Wilkinson, P. C. and Lackie, J. M. (1979). The adhesion, migration and chemotaxis of leucocytes in inflammation. *Curr. Topics in Pathol.* **68**, 48–88.
15. Colditz, I. G. and Movat, H. Z. (1984). Chemotactic factor-specific desensitization of skin to infiltration by polymorphonuclear leukocytes. *Immunol. Lett.* **8**, 83–87.
16. Colditz, I. G. and Movat, H. Z. (1984). Desensitization of acute inflammatory lesions to chemotaxins and endotaxin. *J. Immunol.* **133**, 2163–2168.

17. Colditz, I. G. (1985). Margination and emigration of leucocytes. *Survey & Synthesis in Pathol. Res.* **4**, 44–68.
18. Bevilaqua, M. P., Wheeler, M. E., Pober, J. S., Feirs, W., Mendrick, D. L., Cotran, R. S. and Gimbrone, M. A. (1987). Endothelial-dependent mechanisms of leukocyte adhesion: regulation by interleukin-1 and tumor necrosis factor. *In* "Leukocyte Emigration and its Sequelae" (Ed. H. Z. Movat), 79–93. Karger, Basel.
19. Harlan, J. M., Schwartz, B. R., Willis, W. J. and Pohlman, T. H. (1987). The role of neutrophil membrane proteins in neutrophil emigration. *In* "Leukocyte Emigration and its Sequelae" (Ed. H. Z. Movat), 94–104. Karger, Basel.
20. Colditz, I. G. (1988). Two patterns of early neutrophil accumulation in acute inflammatory lesions. *Inflammation* **12**, 251–263.
21. Cybulsky, M. I., McComb, D. J. and Movat, H. Z. (1988). Protein synthesis dependent and independent mechanisms of neutrophil emigration induced by endotoxin and activated complement. (in press)
22. Colditz, I. G., Kerlin, R. L. and Watson, D. L. (1987). Migration of neutrophils, and their role in elaboration of host defence. *In* "Migration and Homing of Lymphoid cells" (Ed. A. J. Husband). CRC Press, Cleveland. (in press)
23. Lamas, A. M., Mulroney, C. R., Brown, K. E. and Schleimer, R. P. (1987). Studies on the adhesive interaction between human eosinophils and cultured vascular endothelial cells. *Fed. Proc.* **46**, 1041.
24. Archer, C. B., Page, C. P., Paul, W., Morley, J. and MacDonald, D. M. (1983). Early and late inflammatory effects of PAF-acether in the skin of experimental animals and man. *J. Invest. Dermatol.* **80**, 346.
25. McManus, L. M., Hanahan, D. J., Demopoulos, C. A. and Pinckard, R. N. (1980). Pathobiology of the intravenous infusion of acetyl glyceryl ether phosphorylcholine (AGEPC), a synthetic platelet activating factor, in the rabbit. *J. Immunol.* **124**, 2919–2929.
26. Morley, J., Sanjar, S. and Page, C. P. (1985). Pulmonary responses to platelet activating factor. *Prog. Respir. Res.* **19**, 117–123.
27. Arnoux, B., Denjean, A., Page, C. P., Nolibe, D., Morley, J. and Benveniste, J. (1988). Accumulation of platelets and eosinophils in baboon lung following PAF-acether challenge: inhibition by Ketotifen. *Am. Rev. Respir. Dis.* **137**, 855–860.
28. Aoki, S., Boubekeur, K., Burrows, L., Morley, J. and Sanjar, S. (1987). Recruitment of eosinophils by platelet activating factor (PAF) in the guinea-pig lung. *J. Physiol.* **394**, 130P.
29. Border, I., Rogers, S., Chamberlain, D. W., Milne, E. N. C. (1978). Model of allergic bronchoconstriction in the guinea-pig. I. Characteristics of the System. *Clin. Immunopathol.* **9**, 1–15.
30. Hudson, G. (1968). Quantitative study of the eosinophil granulocytes. *Sem. Hematol.* **5**, 166–186.
31. Sabag, N., Castrillon, M. A. and Tchernitchin, A. (1978). Cortisol-induced migration of eosinophil leukocytes to lymphoid organs. *Experientia* **34**, 666–667.
32. Tchernitchin, A. N. and Galand, P. (1983). Oestrogen levels in the blood, not in the endometrium, determine uterine eosinophilia and oedema. *J. of Endocrinol.* **99**, 123–130.
33. Bass, D. A., Gonwa, T. A., Szejda, P., Cousart, M. S., DeChatelet, L. R. and McCall, C. E. (1980). Eosinopenia of acute infection: Production of eosinopenia by chemotactic factors of acute inflammation. *J. Clin. Invest.* **65**, 1265–1271.
34. Lellouch-Tubiana, A., Lefort, J., Pirotzky, E., Vargaftig, B. B. and Pfister, A.

(1985). Ultrastructural evidence for extravascular platelet recruitment in the lung upon intravenous injection of platelet-activating factor (PAF-acether) to guinea-pigs. *Br. J. of Exper. Path.* **66**, 345–355.

35. Zimmerman, G. A., McIntyre, T. M. and Prescott, S. M. (1987). Naturally occurring lipids influence the interaction of human endothelial cells and neutrophils. *In* "Leukocyte Emigration and its Sequelae" (Ed. H. Z. Movat), 105–118. Karger, Basel.

36. Sanjar, S., Morley, J., Page, C. P. and Hanson, J. M. (1987). Platelet activation and airway hyperreactivity in asthma. *In* "Asthma Reviews" (Ed. J. Morley), 1, 141–171.

37. Bewley, J. S. and Chapman, I. D. (1988). AH 21-132 a novel relaxant of airway smooth muscle. *Br. J. Pharmacol.* **93**, 52P.

38. Kristersson, A., Morley, J. and Schaeublin, E. (1988). Properties of AH 21-132 that could contribute to prophylactic activity in asthma. *Br. J. Pharmacol.* **93**, 53P.

39. Spry, C. J. F. (1971). Mechanism of eosinophilia VI. Eosinophil mobilization. *Cell & Tiss. Kin.* **4**, 365–374.

40. Raghavachar, A., Fleischer, A., Frickhofen, N., Heimpel, H. and Fleischer, B. (1987). T lymphocyte control of eosinophilic granulopoiesis. Clonal analysis of an idiopathic hypereosinophilic syndrome. *J. Immunol.* **139**, 3753–3758.

41. Slovick, F. T., Abboud, C. N., Brennan, J. K. and Lichtman, M. A. (1985). Modulation of *in vitro* eosinophil progenitors by hydrocortisone: role of accessory cells and interleukins. *Blood* **66**, 1072–1079.

42. Bjornson, B. H., Harvey, J. M. and Rose, L. (1985). Differential effect of hydrocortisone on eosinophil and neutrophil proliferation. *J. Clin. Invest.* **76**, 28–36.

43. Altman, L. C., Hill, J. S., Hairfield, W. M. and Mullarkey, M. F. (1981). Effects of cortocosteroids on eosinophil chemotaxis and adherence. *J. Clin. Invest.* **67**, 28–36.

44. Keller, H. U. (1985). Granulocyte recruitment and its inhibition. *In* "Handbook of Inflammation, Vol. 5, The Pharmacology of Inflammation" (Eds I. L. Bonta, M. A. Bray and M. J. Parnham), 137–165. Elsevier, Amsterdam.

45. Kay, A. B., Walsh, G. M., Moqbel, R., MacDonald, A. J., Nagakura, T., Carroll, M. P. and Richerson, H. B. (1987). Disodium cromoglycate inhibits activation of human inflammatory cells in vitro. *J. All. & Clin. Immunol.* **80**, 1–8.

46. Diaz, P., Galleguillos, F. R., Gonzales, M. C., Pantin, F. C. A. and Kay, A. B. (1984). Bronchoalveolar lavage in asthma: the effect of disodium cromoglycate (cromolyn) on leukocyte counts, immunoglobulins, and complement. *J. All. & Clin. Immunol.* **74**, 41–48.

47. Dupont, E. and Wybran, J. (1985). Mechanisms of action of corticosteroids. *Int. J. of Immunother.* **1**, 135–138.

48. Braguet, Tougui, P. L., Shen, T. Y. and Vargaftig, B. B. (1987). Perspectives in platelet-activating factor research. *Pharmacol. Rev.* **39**, 97–145.

49. Nakamura, T., Matsumura, Y., Kuriyama, M., Watanabe, A., Ishihara, K., Inokuma, S. and Miyamoto, T. (1987). Ketotifen, an anti-asthmatic drug, inhibits platelet activating factor (PAF) production by human neutrophils. *Proceedings, XII World Congress of Asthmology* 263.

13

Effects of AH21-132 on Bronchial Responses and Eosinophilic Accumulations in the Lungs after Exposure to the Antigen in a Guinea-pig Model of Bronchial Asthma

Y. Terashi, T. Yukawa, S. Motojima and S. Makino

Department of Medicine and Clinical Immunology,
Dokkyo University School of Medicine,
Mibu, Tochigi, 321-02, Japan

13.1 INTRODUCTION

A new anti-asthma drug, AH21-132, was developed by Sandoz Pharmaceuticals (Switzerland). Figure 1 shows the structural Formula of AH21-132. It has been shown that AH21-132 has a bronchodilating potency and inhibits bronchoconstrictions by antigen in sensitized guinea-pigs *in vitro* (Otsuka, T., *et al.* unpublished data).

Eosinophils in Asthma
ISBN 0-12-506452-7

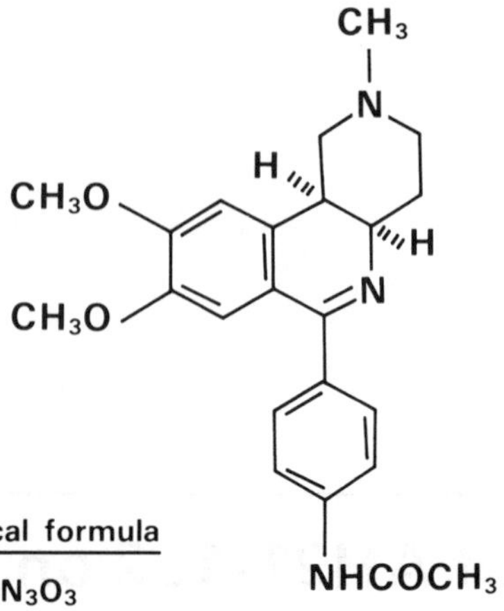

Empirical formula

$C_{23}H_{27}N_3O_3$

Fig. 1   Structural formula of AH21-132.

On the other hand, we have established a model of bronchial asthma using passively sensitized guinea-pigs and found that eosinophils accumulate in bronchial tissues maximally 6 h after antigen challenge (1).

In this experiment, we studied the effects of AH21-132 on pulmonary functions and eosinophilic accumulations in the lungs in the asthmatic model of guinea-pigs.

13.2   MATERIALS AND METHODS

Male Hartley strain guinea-pigs were divided into two groups. One group was injected with 10 mg/kg of AH21-132 intraperitoneally twice a day every day for 2 weeks. The control group was not injected. Guinea-pigs in both groups were passively sensitized to ovalbumin (OA) by injecting 2 ml/kg of anti-OA serum intraperitoneally 48 h before exposure to OA. The serum used for passive immunization was collected from guinea-pigs actively sensitized by repeated injection of OA with alumina gel, with the 48 h passive cutaneous anaphylaxis (PCA) titer of more than 1:640.

One hour after the last injection of AH21-132, an aerosol of 2 mg/ml of OA in saline was administered for 1 min to provoke an allergic bronchoconstriction. Pulmonary functions were recorded for 9 h after antigen challenge.

Pulmonary functions were evaluated by respiratory resistance (Rrs) according to the method by Mead (3) as shown in Figure 2.

The guinea-pigs were sacrificed at 3, 6 and 24 h; the lungs were removed,

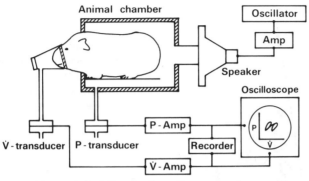

Fig. 2 Schematic illustration of the experimental apparatus for recording of changes of respiratory resistance in guinea-pigs (P, pressure; V̇, flow; Amp, amplifier).

stained by hematoxylin and eosin and Giemsa stain, and used for histological examination.

13.3   RESULTS AND DISCUSSION

The bronchial responses in terms of an increase in Rrs to exposure of OA are shown in Figure 3. Each dot shows the bronchial response of each guinea-pig in the group pretreated by AH21-132. An approximately 3.5-fold increase in Rrs was noticed in the control group. Late asthmatic responses were not recognized in this experimental model. Although the increase in Rrs in the group pretreated by AH21-132 was significantly ($p < 0.001$) lower than that of the control group, the responses of each guinea-pig were diverse. While the increase in Rrs was almost inhibited in about half of the guinea-pigs in the group pretreated by AH21-132, that of other guinea-pigs was not.

The inhibition of the increase in Rrs can be explained by two mechanisms. One is a bronchodilating potency of AH21-132 (Otsuka, T., et al. unpublished data), and the other is that AH21-132 may inhibit the release of chemical mediators by immediate allergic reactions suggested by the fact that AH21-132 can inhibit PCA reaction to some extent (Terashi, Y., et al. unpublished data). However, the mechanisms of bronchodilatation and inhibition of chemical mediator release have not been known.

Plate II a–c shows the histopathology of the lungs obtained 3, 6 and 24 hours, respectively, after OA challenge in the control group stained by Giemsa stain. Almost exclusive accumulations of eosinophils can be recognized in each lung with the peak at 6 hours. Plate II d–f shows the histopatho-

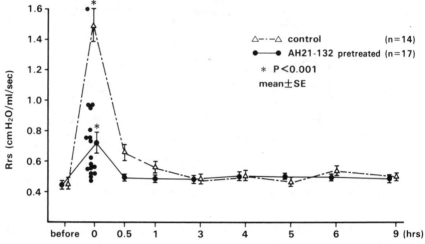

Fig. 3 Time-related changes of the respiratory resistance after exposure to OA in the passively sensitized guinea-pigs with and without pretreatment by AH21-132.

logy of the guinea-pigs pretreated by AH21-132 at 3, 6 and 24 hours, respectively. The accumulations of eosinophils were almost completely inhibited. The findings were almost the same in lung specimens of 2–5 guinea-pigs at each period. The complete blood counts of peripheral blood were normal after the pretreatment by AH21-132 for 14 days. So far the mechanisms of inhibition of eosinophilic accumulations in the lungs are not known. AH21-132 may have other potency than that as a bronchodilator and some inhibiting activities of chemical mediator release.

Although AH21-132 may be a potent drug for a treatment of bronchial asthma because eosinophils accumulated in the lung are suggested to contribute to a worsening and a prolongation of asthmatic attack (4), further studies are needed to elucidate the mechanisms of inhibition of eosinophilic accumulations in the lungs after antigen challenge.

REFERENCES

1. Yukawa, T., Terashi, Y., Fukuda, T. and Makino, S. (1987). Histologic studies on guinea-pig bronchi following inhaled antigen exposure, I. single antigen challenge-induced eosinophilic infiltration and epithelial damage in passively sensitized models (In Japanese). *Jap. J. Allergol.* **36**, 227.
2. Yukawa, T., Makino, S., Fukuda, T. and Kamikawa, Y. (1986). Experimental

model of anaphylaxis-induced β adrenergic blockade in the airways. *Ann. Allergy* **57**, 219.
3. Mead, J. (1960). Control of respiratory frequency. *J. Appl. Physiol.* **15**, 325.
4. Gleich, G. J. and Adolphson, C. R. (1986). The eosinophilic leukocyte: structure and function. *Adv. Immunol.* **39**, 177.

DISCUSSION

Dahl (Chairman): What I make of it is that you see eosinophil infiltration in the bronchi in different experimental systems without having bronchoconstriction. We have seen something similar in human in the nose after allergen challenge, in that we can find increased levels of ECP at 6–8 h, when we would expect a late reaction but without any decrease flow rates in the nose. But after 24 h we see that the nose is more reactive. Have you seen if your animals become hyperreactive?

Sanjar: Certainly. I didn't show the data on actively sensitized animals that were sprayed with antigen. We find a very big eosinophilic response, and at 24 h these guinea-pigs have both depressed basal lung function and they are also hyperreactive to histamine. Eosinophil numbers are elevated at 24, 48 and 72 h and at 1 week after exposure to antigen but the animals are only hyperreactive at 24 and 48 h.

Vadas: Have you taken eosinophils, treated them with PAF, then put them back in the guinea-pig to see if they migrate to the lung?

Sanjar: We have tried to label eosinophils with indium and re-infuse them, and initially they seem to all go to the lung anyway. Separating eosinophils may alter their behaviour somehow, so I can't really answer your question.

Venge: It is difficult to draw conclusions from your experiments with anti-neutrophil serum and anti-platelet serum if you cannot show that there has been complete depletion of these cells from the tissue. Did you look in the lungs for neutrophils for example?

Sanjar: Well, we haven't specifically looked for it, but Dr Holgate's group, who used some of our antisera, have found almost complete absence of neutrophils in the lung and the bronchial washes. So they are fully depleted.

Gleich: Two questions: one for Dr Motojima, and one for Dr Sanjar and Dr Motojima. The first question was on Dr Motojima's experiments. Was bronchial hyperreactivity to histamine or metacholine looked for?

Motojima: In this model using passively sensitized animals we checked the bronchial reactivity to histamine before and 24 h after antigen challenge. Bronchial hyperreactivity seemed to be a little bit higher at 24 h, but the difference was very marginal, with a p value of 0.1.

Gleich: The second question was: do you notice any evidence of epithelial damage?

Sanjar: We have found it quite difficult to quantify epithelial cells in BAL fluid, because they sometimes come in strips and are easy to miss. We are planning to look for epithelial damage.

Gleich: If I recall in the experiments that Paul Kallos reported, initially in German and then later in English, he claimed to see evidence of some desquamation in the guinea-pigs repeatedly nebulized with ovalbumin. Is that your recollection?

Sanjar: Well, that wouldn't really surprise me. Some of these cells we get from antigen-exposed animals are really very damaged. With PAF we see some vacuolated cells and with the antigen challenge we get a lot of dead cells.

Gleich: In other words, in your model it's difficult to make the distinction between dead inflammatory cells or dead epithelial cells?

Sanjar: Yes, it's difficult.

Yukawa: You mentioned that PAF-induced hyperreactivity in guinea-pigs was completely blocked by anti-platelet serum but not by anti-neutrophil serum. However, eosinophil recruitment induced by inhalation of PAF was not inhibited by anti-platelet serum or anti-neutrophil serum. So, could you explain the mechanisms of this discrepancy that anti-platelet serum inhibits PAF-induced hyperreactivity but not PAF-induced eosinophilic infiltration. And the second question is: have you checked the effect of anti-eosinophil serum on both PAF-induced hyperreactivity and eosinophil accumulation?

Sanjar: The first point. Our results suggest that platelets do not play a role in the eosinophilia that follows exposure to PAF. When we give PAF intravenously and the animals are depleted of platelets, they will not give a bronchospasm, but they will give a bronchospasm when you give the PAF challenge by inhalation. So these two routes of administration are quite clearly different for demonstrating the contribution of platelets to PAF-induced bronchoconstriction. As for the second point, you asked about anti-eosinophil serum. In preliminary experiments, our experience has been that we seem to get more eosinophils rather than fewer when we give anti-eosinophil serum. It seems that when depleting eosinophils that are circulating, we somehow switch the animal on to produce many more eosinophils. So, we haven't had the success that we would have hoped for.

Gleich: We've had a lot of experience with anti-eosinophil serum. It's a very, very difficult thing to do. I think we worked five years getting what we thought to be proper anti-eosinophil serum. One thing we did notice though was that with the administration of anti-eosinophil serum, one would deplete the eosinophils in the blood and in the tissues for periods of up to 4 or 5 days. But in some situations, particularly in parasitized animals, doses of anti-eosinophil serum which were adequate to deplete eosinophils in normal guinea-pigs would not be adequate in the animals which had been parasitized. However, we found that in those situations by the simple commonsense pharmacology of giving a larger dose, we were able to deplete eosinophils.

Kay: I have one comment on eosinophils in guinea-pigs and one on PAF inhalation in man. I think as we were saying last night, the guinea-pig is a very eosinophilic type of animal, and it seems to me that really a lot of fairly non-specific manoeuvres can elicit eosinophilia in the guinea-pig. In fact, I think it was you Jerry who pointed out that saline injections into the peritoneal cavity can be associated with profound eosinophilia, so I wonder really how specific this sort of elicitation of eosinophils is in guinea-pigs. With Barnes, Wardlaw and Chang we have been looking at PAF inhalation in man. We haven't gone out as far as you, timewise. Up to 24 h after exposure, we have been more impressed with the neutrophil infiltration in lavage fluid from lungs in normal volunteers inhaling PAF, but those receiving lyso-PAF had relatively few neutrophils. Maybe we would have seen eosinophils if we'd looked a little later.

Venge: Well, I'm just curious about one thing. You say you can inject PAF intravenously, subcutaneously or intraperitoneally and still you find lung eosinophilia. Is this eosinophilia in the lung selective for the lung or do you find it anywhere else in the body? What's the mechanism?

Sanjar: Well, we've looked at bronchial lavages and also peritoneal lavages, and we find that if we give PAF intraperitoneally we get eosinophils in the lungs as we do in the peritoneum. In the peritoneum, there is already quite a substantial resident population of eosinophils which increases following PAF stimulation, so eosinophilia in this instance may be non-specific. We haven't looked in other tissues to know whether, when we induce eosinophilia, these eosinophils are distributed uniformly throughout the animal.

Venge: Do we know if PAF affects the mobilization of eosinophils from bone marrow and affects eosinophilopoiesis.

Sanjar: Well, I should imagine it might be able to do both, but we haven't done those studies.

Makino: I have a comment about PAF-induced bronchial hypersensitivity in man. We have done PAF inhalation or normal subjects and we have found bronchoconstriction immediately after the PAF inhalation. We have found bronchial hypersensitivity to acetylcholine only 1 h after PAF inhalation and not thereafter. So our results differ from Peter Barnes' results. I think PAF-induced bronchoconstriction and bronchial hypersensitivity have two components. And one component is a very early one. One or two hours after the PAF inhalation, in experiments in rabbits, PAF doesn't attract the eosinophils into the bronchi. So probably the early bronchial hypersensitivity induced by PAF is due to oedema of the bronchial mucosa. Bronchial hypersensitivity two or three days later is probably due to eosinophil or some other form of inflammatory cell infiltration. That's my guess.

Capron: I have a comment about the effect of lyso-PAF. Looking at the effect of PAF on increased eosinophil cytotoxicity and increased mediator release, we were surprised to see that lyso-PAF was as effective as PAF on eosinophils. We discussed that result with Jacques Benveniste and he told me that lyso-PAF was clearly ineffective on platelet, but it has not been studied on other cell populations. The current hypothesis is that lyso-PAF in the presence of proper enzymatic equipment is able to induce PAF production by other cells.

14

Allergic Inflammation

J. G. R. de Monchy, E. Kloprogge and H. F. Kauffman

*Department of Allergology,
State University Hospital,
Groningen, The Netherlands*

14.1 INTRODUCTION

Allergy can be described as an immune response directed towards hetero-logous (in principle) not infectious material leading to a (reversible) injury of the host. At the first glance this definition appears permissive because it does not spell out the conditions involved, such as "asthma", allergic rhinitis, skin rash or a drug reaction. This is correct because allergic reactions can involve any organ system in the body. On the other hand, the definition is extremely stringent in that it insists that an immunological mechanism is involved in the pathogenesis and in that auto-immunity, transplantation and tumour-immunity, and the immune response directed against bacteria and viruses are excluded.

Hippocrates (460–377 BC) in his aphorisms mentioned an asthma attack caused by an (at that time unknown) allergic influence. Bostock, in 1819, was

Eosinophils in Asthma
ISBN 0-12-506452-7

the first to describe the symptoms of hay fever. This disease was subsequently known as Bostock's catarrh. In 1873, Blackley discovered that hay fever was caused by pollen (1). As the knowledge concerning allergic reactions increased, the need for a more accurate definition became urgent. It was not until Gell and Coombs made their classification of hypersensitivity reactions that the terminology became unequivocal. Mast cell degranulation caused by reaginic antibodies was subsequently called type I allergy.

Although the identification of IgE as a reaginic antibody greatly enhanced our understanding of allergic diseases, the concept of end organ hyperreactivity was necessary to explain why individuals with the same level of specific IgE may vary in their response to allergen.

14.2   BRONCHIAL HYPERREACTIVITY

Bronchial hyperreactivity can be considered a bronchus obstructive reaction of an individual to stimuli (such as cold air, dust, fog) which, in the majority of the population does not give rise to complaints. Hyperreactivity of the airways is a characteristic feature of the asthmatic patient. The degree of obstruction following an allergic or non-allergic stimulus is dependent on the severity of this stimulus and the degree of airway hyperreactivity. In patients with a high degree of airway hyperreactivity a small stimulus will suffice to cause obstruction. Although there is an association between baseline FEV1 and the degree of bronchial hyperreactivity, bronchial hyperreactivity may vary within certain limits without affecting baseline calibre.

The degree of bronchial hyperreactivity (BH) can be measured with provocation tests. Defined doses of histamine, acetylcholine or metacholine can be inhaled and the response of the bronchi is measured by E.G. spirometry (FEV1).

The degree of BH is correlated to the clinical score of disease (2) and improves in allergic patients during allergen avoidance (3). Since asthmatic patients do not always react in the same degree to stimuli such as cold air, dust and fog, and since for example a viral infection, contact to dust and/or irritants (notably cigarette smoking) may serve as a primer, a more concise definition of bronchial hyperreactivity is needed. One possibility is to consider the measured degree of bronchial hyperreactivity as the sum of a "primary", genetically determined, component, and a "secondary", acquired component. Both on practical and theoretical grounds the distinction between a primary and a secondary component of hyperreactivity is complex. It is conceivable that all hyperreactivity is secondary, but the observation that immunologically similar individuals (with the same degree of specific antibodies) and with a comparable allergen exposition show lasting differences in bronchial hyperreactivity, precludes such an hypothesis. Moreover, patients may be allergic without showing bronchial hyperreactivity or, conversely, may have a marked bronchial hyperreactivity without signs and symptoms of allergy. However BH and IgE *per se* cannot explain the presence or absence of late allergic reactions, and a "third factor" must be postulated (4). This third factor is possibly associated with the fact that, during inhalation, provocation biphasic bronchial obstructive reactions are followed by an increase in peripheral eosinophil counts, while patients who only have an early phase reaction lack this increase (5).

14.3 LATE ALLERGIC REACTIONS

Late allergic reactions have been documented in various tissues such as the skin (7), the lungs (8), and the nasal mucosa (9), of sensitized subjects.

Although single late allergic reactions occasionally occur, the late reaction is classically the second part of a biphasic response. While the early phase occurs some 15 min following an allergen contact, and subsides within 1 h, the late phase starts about 3 h after allergen contact, reaches its maximum after 7–8 h, and may still be present after 24 h.

The mechanism of the early phase was shown to be dependent on IgE mediated mast cell (or basophil) degranulation, but the mechanism of the late phase is largely unknown.

Patients who exhibit a biphasic response following allergen challenge seem to have a more serious type of bronchial "asthma" than those who have single early reactions (EAR) (8). This may be related to the observation that the LAR may induce an increase in bronchial hyperreactivity (10).

The clinical pattern of the EAR and the LAR are not identical. The LAR is of longer duration than the EAR and does not react as readily to β-agonists as the EAR does (11). In contrast to the EAR, pretreatment with corticosteroids usually abolishes the LAR (12). Also non-steroidal anti-inflammatory drugs may offer protection against the development of the LAR (13). The LAR was also shown recently to be responsive to xanthine derivatives (14). Because of its typical occurrence 3–8 h after inhalation of allergen, an IgG-immune complex mediated reaction was originally suggested by Pepys to explain the mechanism of the LAR (15). The generation of immune complexes of IgG with inhaled antigen, and subsequent activation of the complement cascade by the classic route with production of anaphylatoxins C3a and C5a, was suggested as a means of inducing mast cell degranulation resulting in a second phase of bronchial obstruction largely independent of IgE antibodies.

This hypothesis was mainly evaluated by studying the late response in the skin of patients with bronchopulmonary aspergillosis (ABPA). But the mould-induced skin or bronchial reaction does not seem to be a good model to study HDM-induced LAR.

14.4 BRONCHOALVEOLAR LAVAGE FOLLOWING HDM CHALLENGE

In patients with a LAR a local bronchoalveolar eosinophilia was found. This eosinophilia was not present in patients who had only experienced an EAR when lavage was carried out 6–7 h after allergen inhalation (16). Moreover, when BAL was carried out 2–3 h after bronchial challenge in patients who had previously been shown to develop a LAR, no eosinophilia was present. In the LAR group, the bronchoalveolar eosinophilia was accompanied by a rise in the eosinophil cationic protein (ECP) in the BAL fluid. This probably indicated an increased metabolic activity of these cells. No evidence was found for neutrophil infiltration during the LAR, neither by the analysis of differential cell counts, by detection of lactoferrin, a neutrophil-derived substance, nor by measurement of lysozyme, which may be produced by neutrophils or alveolar macrophages in addition to some production by mucous glands (17). It is known that eosinophil cells, in contrast to neutrophil granulocytes, produced the spasmogenic LTC_4 upon stimulation with serum treated Zymosan (STZ). Since asthmatic patients have been shown to be hypersensitive to leukotrienes (18), infiltration of eosinophils and activation of these cells may be crucial to the development of the LAR.

As the eosinophil was shown to be the main infiltrating cell in asthma (19), and since Frigas (20) showed that in the sputum of patients with asthma exacerbations the eosinophil derived major basic protein (MBP) was strongly elevated, the LAR may serve as a laboratory model for day-to-day asthma.

The clinical pattern of the LAR is quite different from the EAR, but major biochemical differences also can be found. As shown previously, the EAR is not accompanied by cell infiltration but seems to be strongly mediator-dependent. We found rises in urinary Nt-methylhistamine following the EAR, indicating production of histamine during the EAR but, during the LAR, no increase in urinary Nt-methylhistamine was found (21, 22). In bronchoalveolar lavage fluid of LAR patients, higher histamine levels were found than in the other patient groups. Since histamine in the BAL-fluid may be derived from mechanical injury to mast cells the histamine metabolite Nt-methyl-histamine was measured which is a better parameter for histamine production *in vivo* than histamine itself (22). In the LAR group, Nt-methylhistamine was not different from controls. This suggests that, although some histamine may be produced during the LAR, histamine probably is not the main mediator substance (17).

Togias *et al.* (23) found during the late reaction in the nose, histamine, kinins, kininogens and leukotrienes. During the early reaction the same mediators were found, but also prostaglandin D_2. Since prostaglandin D_2 is mast cell-dependent, the absence of the latter mediator during the LAR may indicate that histamine elevation during the LAR may not be derived from mast cells but from other histamine-containing cells such as basophil granulocytes. During the late reaction, basophils could be attracted by chemotactic substances and produce mediators directly by binding IgE and allergen to their surface. Histamine release could also occur by intervention of eosinophils in an IgG-dependent fashion since cationic proteins increase basophil releasability (24).

The question remains, how the eosinophil is "drawn" into the allergic process. This could happen as a result of chemotactic stimulation by mast cells, alveolar macrophages or other cells.

One of the most potent eosinophil chemotactic substances present, is platelet activating factor (PAF). PAF can be derived from mast cells, but also from the alveolar macrophages, in much larger amounts present in the lung. Alveolar macrophages (AM) have IgE receptors, thus also the IgE dependence of the LAR could be explained. Neutrophil chemotactic activity (NCA), clearly elevated during both EAR and LAR, can be derived from AMs but also from mast cells. However, since NCA was found to be of the high molecular type (HMW)-NCA, the mast call origin is likely (25). Plasma HMW-NCA rise following allergen challenge was recently shown to coincide with a rise in two molecular weight eosinophil chemotactic factors LMW-ECF (26) which could also be derived from mast cells or from macrophages.

14.5 ALTENARIA

Metzger and co-workers, performing a bronchoalveolar lavage before and 4 and 24 h after an Altenaria allergen provocation in allergic asthmatics, observed that the number of eosinophils was already elevated 4 h after the inhalation test and was still significantly increased after 24 h. The number of neutrophils appears to be increased after 4 h, but not after 24 h. Transmission electron microscope studies of the lavage fluid showed evidence of degranulation of mast cells and eosinophils (27).

14.5.1   Toluene Diisocyanate (TDI)

Like allergens such as house dust mite, TDI can induce both an early and/or late asthmatic response in sensitized subjects. An early response after exposure to TDI is thought to be due to bronchial smooth muscle contraction, because it can be reversed by a bronchodilator. A late asthmatic response induced by TDI is, however, not prevented by a bronchodilator but only by corticosteroids. Fabbri and co-workers (28) found in the bronchoalveolar lavage fluid in subjects with late asthmatic responses on TDI exposure, an increased number of neutrophils at both 2 and 8 h, whereas eosinophils were only increased at 8 h.

After having assessed an increase of bronchial reactivity after TDI exposure in 5 subjects showing a late asthmatic reaction to TDI, Fabbri and co-workers studied the effects of prednisolone and indomethacin on this reaction. Prednisolone inhibited both the late asthmatic reaction and the increase in bronchial hyperreactivity, while treatment with indomethacin showed no effect on either phenomenon (28). Since corticosteroids are believed to influence the arachidonic acid cascade and indomethacin is known to inhibit the cyclooxygenase pathway, it seems likely that the lipooxygenase metabolites play a role in the development of late allergic reaction after TDI exposure.

14.5.2   Red Cedar

Plicatic acid is the compound responsible for red cedar asthma. Exposure can induce both an early and/or a late asthmatic response. Lam and co-workers carried out a bronchoalveolar lavage at different time intervals in patients known to show a late asthmatic response to this agent (29). These investigators observed a significant increase in the number of eosinophils within 2 h after the provocation test and this number remained elevated at 24 h. The proportion of neutrophils became elevated after 48 h. In the patients also bronchial biopsies were performed and showed a marked damage of the bronchial epithelium.

14.5.2.1   In vitro studies of eosinophil activation

Thus in many models of allergic inflammation eosinophils were shown to be present and probably play a causative role in the development of the LAR. Morphologic characteristics of BAL cells seem to indicate that these cells are in the so-called hypodense state.

These hypodense cells were described as "activated" eosinophils, with respect to killing properties, oxygen radical production, receptor expression and leukotriene production (30, 31, 32, 33).

In vitro studies of purified eosinophils offer the possibility to compare characteristics of normodense and hypodense cells of asthmatic patients, with those of non-atopic, healthy individuals. Proper investigations of normal eosinophils require a reliable way of isolation of eosinophils from blood of normals. Till now, however, most studies have used eosinophils obtained from patients with eosinophilia.

A recent publication described a method to isolate eosinophils under optimal conditions (34). Using this method we found over 90% of the isolated eosinophils with a density between 1.095 and 1.105 g/ml in the blood of normal healthy volunteers. These cells were defined as normodense eosinophils (35). Eosinophils with a lower density < 1.095 g/ml were named hypodense cells. Compared to Fukuda *et al.* (36), the average of densities of the eosinophils from normal non-atopic persons was about 0.010–0.015 g/ml higher. The differences in densities, as also reported by other authors, may be explained by the isotonic isolation procedure at a lower pH of 7.0 and/or the avoidance of glassware and vacuum systems during blood collection, to avoid activation of blood platelets. In agreement with other reports (31, 36, 37), an increased percentage of hypodense eosinophils in the peripheral blood of patients with atopic asthma was found.

In our study, 7 of the patients were in a stable phase of their disease, as reflected by absence of bronchial obstruction and normal eosinophil counts. Three other patients showed hypereosinophilia. The density distribution of the eosinophils in the atopic asthmatic patients showed 65% hypodense cells, as defined by the distribution pattern found in a normal group. Although the total amount of hypodense eosinophils was increased in patients with hypereosinophilia, the ratio hypodense/normodense eosinophils was similar to the patients with normal cell counts.

There have been many speculations on the generation of hypodense eosinophils found in patients with eosinophilia of different origin. We therefore wondered if hypodense eosinophils could be raised *in vitro*, by activation of purified normodense eosinophils. Stimulation of normodense eosinophils, isolated from blood samples of the healthy non-atopic volunteers, induced a remarkable shift from normodense to hypodense density for a number of stimuli, except for fMLP (Table 1).

As a parameter of cell activation, the O_2-production was measured with

Table 1 Percentage of hypodense eosinophils induced by stimulation of normodense eosinophils *in vitro*. (Data are expressed as means ± SD)

Stimulator	Percentage of shift to hypodense < 1.095 g/ml	Number of experiments
controls	< 5%	2
fMLP	7.8 ± 12.0	4
STZ	64.5 ± 13.6	3
A23187	74.5 ± 16.3	7
PAF-acether	52.8 ± 17.0	5

the same cell populations as described in Table 2. Activation of normodense eosinophils was performed with the same stimuli. Non-stimulated eosinophils showed a spontaneous O_2-production of 1.7 nmol cytochrome C reduction when incubated for 15 min at 37°C. Stimulation of the cells resulted in a significant increase of the O_2-production. A23187 turned out to be the most potent stimulus for O_2-production, followed by STZ and PAF-acether (35). The potency of those stimuli in raising hypodense eosinophils was in the same order, A23187 > STZ > PAF-acether (35). fMLP, at a concentration of 2×10^{-8} M, was less potent in the stimulation of O_2-production and did not induce any shift from normodense to hypodense eosinophils. STZ was confirmed by microscopic analysis to be phagocytosed.

These data show that a physiological stimulus as PAF-acether, that may be derived from an IgE mediated process induces eosinophils to become activated.

14.6 CONCLUSION

Allergic inflammation is now widely accepted to be one of the important causes of bronchial "asthma", although the nature of this inflammation,

Table 2 Superoxide production of normodense eosinophilic granulocytes after 15 min incubation and stimulation at 37°C, expressed as the amount of cytochrome C reduction (means ± SD; p values with a student's t-test, $n = 6$).

Stimulator	nmol cytochrome C reduction in 15 min per 10^6 cells	p value compared to control
control	1.71 ± 0.34	
fMLP	3.2 ± 1.9	< 0.01
STZ	6.3 ± 1.8	< 0.01
A23187	7.5 ± 3.2	< 0.01
PAF-acether	3.7 ± 2.4	< 0.03

depending on the provoking factors, may be different. Many questions remain, one of the most intriguing ones is whether granulocytes are directly linked to tissue injury and inflammation. Recent work of Venge and co-workers and Gleich has shown that eosinophils indeed have a huge potential for tissue injury (39, 40). In our studies, using house dust mite allergen, no direct or indirect evidence was found for the involvement of neutrophil cells in allergic inflammation but other antigens, such as fungi or chemical substances such as TDI, may trigger neutrophil responses. However, the studies performed by Metzger and Fabbri (26–28), concerning these substances showed eosinophil infiltration as well as neutrophilia.

A second point is—what attracts cells to the site of the allergic response? The attraction of eosinophils could be the result of mast cell degranulations, since Kay has already shown in 1971 that, following IgE-mediated stimulation and eosinophil leukocyte chemotactic factor was liberated from human lung (low molecular weight eosinophil chemotactic factor) (41). Several chemotactic substances for eosinophils both heat labile and heat stabile have been detected. Until now however it was not known with certainty from which cell these substances are mainly derived (42).

Allergic (eosinophilic) inflammation may be the "missing link" between IgE and the signs and symptoms of asthma.

REFERENCES

1. Blackley, C. H. (reprint 1959). Experimental researches on the cause and nature of catarrhas aestivas. Dowsons of Pall Mall, London 1873.
2. Cockroft, D. W., Killian, D. N., Metton, J. J. A. and Hargreave, F. E. (1977). Bronchial reactivity to inhaled histamine a method and clinical survey. *Clin. Allergy* 7, 235–243.
3. Platts-Mitts, T. A. E., Mitohd, E. B. and Nock, P. (1982). Reduction of bronchial hyperreactivity during prolonged allergen avoidance. *Lancet II*, 675–678.
4. Monchy de J. G. R. (1986). The late allergic reaction in bronchial asthma. Thesis, Groningen Krips Repro.
5. Booy Noord, A., Vries, K. de, Sluiter, H. J. and Orie, N. G. M. (1972). Late bronchial obstructive reaction to experimental inhalation of house dust extract. *Clin. Allergy* 2, 43–61.
6. Monchy de, J. G. R., Kauffman, H. F., Venge, P, Koëter, G. H., Kansen, H. M., Sluiter, H. J., Vries, K. de (1983). Broncho alveolar eosinophilia during allergen induced late asthmatic reactions. *Am. Rev. Resp. Dis.* 131, 373–376.
7. Cooke, R. A. (1922). Studies in specific hypersensitiveness. XI. On the phenomenon of hyposensitiveness, (The clinical lessened sensitiveness of allergy). *J. Immunol.* 7, 219.
8. Herxheimer, H. (1952). The late bronchial reaction in induced asthma. *Int. Arch. Allergy Appl. Immunol.* 3, 323–328.

9. Taylor, G and Shivalkar, P. R. (1971). Arthus type reactivity in the nasal airways and skin in pollen sensitive subjects. *Clin. Allergy* **1**, 407–414.
10. Cartier, A., Frith, P. H. Roberts, R., Thomson, N. C. and Hargreave F. E. (1982). Allergen induced increased in bronchial responsiveness to histamine: relationship to the late asthmatic response and change in airway caliber. *J. Allergy Clin. Immunol.* **70**, 170–177.
11. Booy-Noord, H., Quanjer, Ph. H. and Vries, K. de (1972). Protektive wirkung von Berotec bei provokations Testen mit Specifischer Allergen Inhalation und Histamin. *Int. J. Clin. Pharmacol.* **4**, 69–72.
12. Booy-Noord, H., Orie, N. G. M. and Vries, K. de (1971). Immediate and late Bronchial obstructive reactions to inhalation of house dust and protective affect disodium cromoglycate and prednisolon. *J. Allergy Clin. Immunol.* **48**, 344–354.
13. Fairfax, A. J., Hanson, J. M. and Morley, J. (1983). The late reaction following bronchial provocation with house dust mite allergen. Dependence on arachidonic acid metabolism. *Clin. Exp. Immunol.* **52**, 393–398.
14. Pauwels, R., Rentergem, D. van, Straeten, M. van der, Johannesson, N. and Persson C. G. A. (1985). The effect of theophylline and enprohylline on allergen; induced bronchoconstriction. *J. Allergy Clin. Immunol.* **76**, 583–590.
15. Dolovich, J., Hargreave, F. E., Chalmers, R., Shier, K. J., Gauldie, J. and Bienenstock, J. (1973). Late cutaneous allergic responses in isolated IgE dependent reactions. *J. Allergy Clin. Immunol.* **52**, 38–46.
16. Monchy, J. G. R. de, Kauffman, H. F., Venge, P., Koëter, G. H., Janssen, H. M., Sluiter, H. J. and Vries, K. de (1985) Broncho alveolar eosinophilia during allergen induced late asthmatic reactions. *Am. Rev. Resp. Dis.* **131**, 373–376.
17. Monchy, J. G. R. de (1985). The late asthmatic reaction in bronchial asthma. Thesis. Krips repro Meppel.
18. Adelroth, R., Morris, M. M., Hargreave, F. E. and O'Byrne, P. M. (1986). Airway responsiveness to leukotrienes C_4 and D_4 and to metacholine in patients with asthma and normal controls. *N. Engl. J. Med.* **315**, 480–484.
19. Dunhill, M. S. (1975). The morphology of the airways in bronchial asthma. *In* "New Directions in Asthma" (Ed. M. Stein), 213. American College of chest physicians. Park Ridge, Illinois.
20. Frigas, R., Dor, P. J. and Gleich, G. J. (1983). The usefulness of sputum radioimmuno assay for the eosinophil major basic protein in the diagnosis of asthma. *Folia Allergol. Immun. Pathol.* **30** (4), 92.
21. Monchy, J. G. R. de, Keijzer, J. J., Kauffman, H. F., Beaumont, F. and Vries, K. de (1985). Histamine in late asthmatic reactions following house dust mite inhalation. *Agents & Actions* **16**, 225.
22. Keijzer, J. J., Kauffman, H. F., Monchy, J. G. R. de, Keijzer-Udding, J. J. and Vries K. de (1984) Urinary Nt-methylhistamine during early and late allergen induced bronchial obstructive reactions. *J. Allergy Clin. Immunol.* **74**, 240–245.
23. Togias, A., Naclerio, R. M., Proud, D., Baumgarten, C., Peters, S., Creticos, P. S., Warner, J., Kagey Sobotka, A., Adkinison, N., Norman, P. S. and Lichtenstein, L.M. (1985). Mediator release during nasal provocation, a model to investigate the pathophysiology of rhinitis. *Am. J. Med.* **79** (6A), 26–32.
24. O'Donne, M. C., Ackerman, S. J., Gleich, G. J. and Thomas, L. L. (1982). Activation of basophil and mast cell histamine release by eosinophil granula major basic protein. *J. Exp. Med.* **157**, 1981–1989.
25. Nagy, I., Lee, T. H., Goetzl, E. J., Pickett, W.. and Kay, A. (1982). Neutrophil

chemotactic activity in antigen induced late asthmatic reactions. *N. Engl. J. Med.* **305**, 497–501.

26. Metzger, W. J., Richerson, H. B. and Wasserman, S. I. (1986). Generation of and partial characterization of eosinophil chemotactic activity and neutrophil chemotactic activity during early and late phase asthmatic response. *J. Allergy Clin. Immunol.* **78**, 282–290.

27. Metzger, W. J., Richerson, H. B., Worden, B. S., Marick, M. and Hunninghake, G. W. (1986). Broncho alveolar lavage of allergic asthmatic patients following allergen provocation. *Chest* **89**, 477–483.

28. Fabbri, L., Di Giacomo, R., Vecchio. K., Zocca, E., De Marro, N., Meastralli, P. and Mapp, C. E. (1985). Prednisone, indomethacin and airway responsiveness in Toluene Diisocyanate sensitized subjects. *Clin. Respir. Phys.* **21**, 421–426.

29. Lam, S., Leriche, J., Philips, D. and Chan-Yeung, M. (1987). Cellular and protein changes in bronchial lavage fluid after late asthmatic reaction in patients with red cedar asthma. *J. Allergy Clin. Immunol.* **80**, 44–50.

30. Butterworth, A. E., Sturrock, R. F., Houba, V., Mahmoud, A. A. F., Sher, A. and Rees, P. K. (1975). Eosinophils as mediators of antibody-dependent damage to schistosomula. *Nature* **256**, 727–729.

31. Kauffman, H. F., Belt, B. van der, Monchy, J. G. R. de, Boelens, H. Koëter, G. H. and Vries, K. de (1987). Leukotriene C_4 production by normal density and low-density eosinophils of atopic individuals and other patients with eosinophilia. *J. Allergy Clin. Immunol.* **79**, 611–619.

32. Spry, J. F. (1985). Synthesis and secretion of eosinophil granula substances. *Immunol. Today* **6**, 332–335.

33. Simone, C. de, Donelli, G., Meli, D., Rosati, F. and Sorci F. (1982). Human eosinophils and parasitic diseases. II. Characterization of two cell fractions isolated at different densities. *Clin. Exp. Immunol.* **48**, 249–255.

34. Yazdanbakhsh, M., Eckmann, C. M., Boer, M. de and Roos, D. (1987). Purification of eosinophils from normal human blood, preparation of eosinoplasts and characterization of their functional response to various stimuli. *Immunology* **60**, 123–129.

35. Kloprogge, E., Leeuw, A. J. de Monchy, J. G. R. de and Kauffman, H. F. (1989). Hypodense eosinophilic granulocytes in normal individuals and patients with asthma: generation of hypodense cell populations in vitro. *J. Allergy Clin. Immunol.* **83**, 393.

36. Fukuda, T., Dunnette, S. L., Reed, C. E., Ackerman, S. J., Peters, M. S. and Gleich G. J. (1985). Increased numbers of hypodense eosinophils in the blood of patients with bronchial asthma. *Am. Rev. Respir. Dis.* **123**, 981–985.

37. Kauffman, H. F., Belt, B. van der, Monchy, J. G. R. de, Boelens, H., Koëter, G. H. and Vries, K. de (1987). Leucotriene C_4 production by normal density and low-density eosinophils of atopic individuals and other patients with eosinophilia. *J. Allergy Clin. Immunol.* **79**, 611–619.

38. Dahl, R. and Venge, P. (1982). Role of the eosinophil in bronchial asthma. *Eur. J. Respir. Dis.* **122**, 23–28.

39. Venge, P., Dahl, R., Fredens, K., Hällgren, R. and Peterson, C. (1983). Eosinophil cationic proteins (ECP and EPX) in health and disease. *In* "Immunobiology of the Eosinophil" (Eds T. Yochida and M. Torisu), 163–179. North Holland, Amsterdam.

40. Gleich, G. J., Frigas, E., Loegering, D. A., Wassom, D. L. and Steinmuller, D.

(1979). Cytotoxic properties of the eosinophil major basic protein. *J. Immunol.* **123**, 2925–2927.
41. Kay, A. B. and Austen, F. R. (1971). The IgE mediated release of an eosinophil leucocyte chemotactic factor from human lung. *J. Immunol.* **107**, 899–902.
42. Rak, S. (1988). Bronchial hyperresponsiveness and cellular and humoral factors involved in allergic inflammation during pollen season. Thesis, Lund, Sweden.

DISCUSSION

Dahl (Chairman): I think it may be sometimes difficult to say when a late reaction is present.

Kay: Yes, I agree with you that one has to resist the temptation to categorize patients very rigidly into two groups. The cut-off point is 25% fall in the FEV_1 during the late phase reaction and we tried as far as possible to take the two ends of the spectrum.

Gleich: If I understand correctly, Dr de Monchy, in the first study you performed you showed only eosinophils increasing in the BAL, that there had been a prior antigen challenge a week before?

de Monchy: Yes, that's right.

Gleich: In your lavages, did you look for mast cells?

de Monchy: Well, we looked for them, but we found very low frequencies and found it very difficult to quantify them, so we didn't do that. We found very low counts.

Wasserman: Did you measure histamine?

de Monchy: Yes, we measured histamine. We found no significant differences in histamine from the patient group, but we looked also at methylhistamine and there we found a trend to higher levels, but it was not very impressive.

Gleich: And one last point. These are difficult experiments to do, but it would seem to me that in some of these experiments one should consider the possibility of additional controls, for example, giving the antigen which you used to challenge the asthmatics to patients who are not sensitive and giving the patients an unrelated antigen to which they are not sensitive. In other words, you need to be really sure that the cell infiltration that you are observing is related because there is potential for, it seems to me, much mischief here.

de Monchy: Well, if you really want to select on the basis of IgE-mediated responses, and of course that's what we want, then it would be worthwhile. On the other hand, as you mentioned, it is a very complicated type of investigation and it takes a lot of the patient to say to him, well we challenge you now with cat and dog and birch. But basically you're right, I think.

Gleich: In fairness, I should say that I'm making this comment as someone from outside the arena. I appreciate the complications that you experience in attempting to do this.

Kay: I think it really depends on the question you're asking. If you're comparing dual responders and single early responders, as we were, I think that is a big enough question to ask in this sort of study. There is a major problem of choosing an unrelated antigen in the whole context of aero-allergens and also of distinguishing between non-specific bronchial hyperreactivity induced by the putative non-cross-reacting antigen and knowing what dose range to be in. So there are formidable problems there.

Gleich: Just one other point. It's said that after a late reaction and this comes out of Hargrave's group and I think Cartier is the first author of the paper, that following a late reaction there is an increase in bronchial hyperreactivity. But recently I was forced to go back and I appreciated from examining the data rather more carefully that the patients who did not have late reactions, but who had antigen challenge, also had increases in bronchial hyperreactivity which were almost as great as the patients who had the late reactions. I thought this was rather intriguing and in light of Barry's observations where the changes in these cells recovered by BAL in a tendency to be significant.

Kay: A number of studies, particularly the one by Durham and Taylor, showed that this change in reactivity in fact comes before the late phase reaction. In fact you can show this change in reactivity at 3 h after antigen challenge, and it's those patients who react who will then go on to the late phase reaction. So it's really the other way around.

Gleich: What do you mean it's the other way around?

Kay: Well, it's not the late-phase reaction causing the hyperreactivity, it's the hyperreactivity causing the late-phase reaction.

de Monchy: Well, I object to that, Barry, I don't think you can say it.

Kay: Well, I was overstating the case just to put the point across very briefly. It's more complicated.

Gleich: But, one last point and that is, if one does biopsies of cutaneously late-phase reactions, you can see striking eosinophil and neutrophil degranulation by $1\frac{1}{2}$ h.

de Monchy: Yes, I know that. There is the question of to what degree does the bronchial lavage represent what is happening in the interstitium. Ideally, you should try to get some biopsies, but that's quite complicated, and patients are not happy to co-operate after they've coughed up some blood.

Dahl: After 2 h you had increases in your ECP levels in the lavage fluid?

de Monchy: Yes, there was some increase in ECP level.

Wasserman: I was just going to make a cautionary point. I think that these are interesting observations, it's hard to call them experiments in a way because we don't know what the hypothesis is often and what we are testing. What concerns me is when we begin to get a list of 30 and 40 different things we are observing and measuring and we don't know the interrelationships between those measurements. For example, if you are going to measure ECP and MBP and EDN they ought to be correlated, we are going to get families of correlations that don't mean anything. And if you measure 20 or 30 things and ask for a .05 level of significance, one or two of them are going to be significant, statistically but not biologically, just because you measured so many things. It's not a criticism, it's just a cautionary note. I think Barry was overstating the case but, I think it's extremely important not to assume that because we see something that there is any causative relationship between what we see in one area and what we observe in another. I mean, causation here is completely obscure.

de Monchy: The first point you made is that you would like to see a correlation between all these mediators and I think during the whole morning session we have been focusing upon differences.

Wasserman: I'm saying that if you measure so many things and look for correlation, we are going to come up with correlations that are mathematical correlations but are biologically meaningless.

de Monchy: Well, I must object to that point strongly. In the lavage studies we just measured cells and ECP and there was an hypothesis behind it; it was not King correlation reigning again. There are many studies now suggesting the importance of eosinophils on bronchial hyperreactivity and baseline lung function, so these parameters were not selected in a random way but were implicated. I showed you the scheme which we adhere to and where we try to fill in the gaps.

Wasserman: I'm not being critical of your experiments at all. I'm being critical of the leap to causation, because we haven't a clue about causation.

de Monchy: Of course you're right.

Wasserman: And in fact they may only be correlated to some other truly important phenomena that we don't know how to measure yet.

de Monchy: Well, of course, you're right.

Dahl: You've made a new observation and made your hypothesis and are going to test it now in future experiments. Do you think there is anything in the selection of patients that influences the results.

de Monchy: Well, we looked at one segment of the asthmatic population. If you pick out 20 asthmatic patients from the clinic, you might get a different picture. I think it's necessary to keep the group somewhat clean and therefore we looked at patients who were non-smokers, who were in hospital, who had no recent infections, etc.

Wasserman: It is extremely important that we remember that the bronchoalveolar lavage fluid is probably not where the action is taking place, it is what's left over and may be totally unrepresentative of what's going on within the tissue of the lung. Now, I grant you that if it's hard to get bronchoalveolar lavage performed, so is it going to be a little more difficult to do lung biopsies on all these patients. But perhaps that's really where we ought to be and what we're seeing in the lavage may be the tip of the iceberg or may be a totally eroneous area to be looking at. It might be analogous to looking at the blood instead of the joint in rheumatoid arthritis.

Spry: There have now been I think about 18 published reports on broncho-alveolar lavage in asthmatic patients either without challenge or with challenge, and you've beautifully reviewed many of the important ones for us. What do you think is the next step in this area of respiratory pathophysiology? Do you think you have now established that there is a sufficiently clear-cut picture of the cellular changes that occur or do you think that some of the earlier work needs to be repeated in the light of the new discoveries you've made about the changes that occur? I would like as an outsider to know the emphasis you'd like to put on bronchoalveolar lavage in asthma reasearch at the moment. It's rather a large question, but I'd be interested to know what sort of experiments you would recommend others to do, because there are many different groups around the world who are picking up your skills and would wish to apply them.

de Monchy: Well, I think that bronchoalveolar lavage can be done if you have done prior studies which give the basis for such an experiment. I don't think it should be used as a screening method for the effectiveness of drugs or if you have some faint ideas of mechanisms. I think we should also look very much at the use of more advanced lung function techniques which perhaps can differentiate effects of bronchoconstriction and bronchodilation versus the inflammatory effects. On the other hand, you can use cells harvested from BAL fluid to do many experiments after first learning the techniques on blood cells. I think lavage should be used as a more advanced step in the assessment of mechanisms, drug actions, etc.

Spry: So, you recommend the cellular studies as being the most useful ones not the mediator assays, is that right?

de Monchy: Yes, I think as far as you can differentiate between these things, yes.

Bruijnzeel: Has anyone any ideas about the ratio of hypodense to normo-dense eosinophils in various tissues after antigen challenge?

Dahl: I think we have to end this session with this intriguing question which we may solve, not in the coffee break but hopefully before the next meeting. Thank you very much, de Monchy.

15

Eosinophil Lipid Mediators and Granule Secretory Products in Allergy and Asthma

A. B. Kay, A. J. Frew, R. Moqbel, G. M. Walsh, K. Kurihara, O. Cromwell, A. Champion, A. Hartnell and A. J. Wardlaw

Department of Allergy and Clinical Immunology, National Heart & Lung Institute, London SW3 6LY UK

15.1 INTRODUCTION

Eosinophils are a hallmark of IgE-mediated allergic diseases. They infiltrate the tissue in large numbers in the skin, nose and bronchi after allergen challenge in sensitized atopic subjects. Many appear to be degranulated and it is believed that eosinophil products, particularly granule-associated basic proteins and membrane-derived lipids, may be directly responsible for tissue damage (especially epithelial shedding and mucous hypersecretion which is

Eosinophils in Asthma
ISBN 0-12-506452-7

characteristic of allergic inflammation at mucosal surfaces). Over the past few years our group, and others, have studied the phenomenon of eosinophil activation, both *in vitro* and *in vivo*. The *in vitro* experiments have attempted to increase our knowledge of the eosinophil's repertoire in terms of its responsiveness to pharmacological mediators, particularly those acting through receptors for IgE (FcεRII), IgG (Fc) and complement. The *in vivo*, clinical studies were undertaken to provide evidence that eosinophil activation (as shown by the presence of secreted granule products) was related to clinical manifestations and that this in turn might offer further insight into pathogenetic mechanisms, particularly in allergy and asthma.

Over the past decade or so several groups have studied the heterogeneity of human peripheral blood eosinophils. In particular, it is now appreciated that cells obtained from patients with hypereosinophilia are metabolically more active than normal eosinophils (1) and separate into low, as well as normal, density cells after centrifugation on Percoll or Metrizamide gradients (2–4). It is now clear that at least a proportion of these low density cells represent a subpopulation of activated cells. For instance, in the same individual low density cells have increased expression of Fcγ (3) and Fcε receptors (5), are more cytotoxic for opsonised helminths *in vitro* (6), produce more LTC_4 than normodense cells after incubation with IgG-coated beads (7) and, in general, respond more vigorously in chemotaxis (8). Low-density cells also showed complete or partial loss of the crystalline granule core and, in this sense, probably correspond to the vacuolated cells previously observed in peripheral blood from patients with the hypereosinophilic syndrome (9). In the tissues, activated cells can be recognized by a monoclonal antibody (EG2) which distinguishes between the storage and secreted forms of the eosinophil cationic protein (ECP) (10).

The T cell dependence of control of eosinophilia in rodents has been recognized since the early 1970s and there is now a sizeable literature on eosinophil maturation and activation by various cytokines (reviewed in 11). It has been shown that tumour necrosis factor (TNF), granulocyte/macrophage-colony stimulating factor, IL-3 and IL-5 can augment eosinophil function in a number of ways, including enhanced cytotoxic capacity, up-regulation of membrane markers and increased metabolic activity (12, 13). In our experience, resting human eosinophils, unlike neutrophils, respond weakly in directional locomotion (chemotaxis) to a wide range of cytokines, including IL-5, even when tested over a wide concentration range (14). In contrast, platelet activating factor (PAF) is a potent eosinophil chemo-attractant and, as described below, activates eosinophils to a comparable degree to LTB_4. Furthermore, a variety of physiological stimuli lead to relatively large amounts of both PAF and LTC_4 generation by eosinophils.

15.2   PAF AND EOSINOPHIL CHEMOTAXIS

Platelet activating factor (1-0-alkyl-2-acetyl-*sn*-glycero-3-phosphocholine) is a potent inflammatory mediator with a wide range of biological activities (reviewed in 15). In human tissues these activities include platelet aggregation and secretion, bronchoconstriction and induction of non-specific bronchial hyperreactivity, leucocyte chemotaxis, modulation of cellular immune functions and inflammatory changes in the skin.

There is comparatively little information on eosinophil activation by PAF. In a previous study we showed that PAF induced directional locomotion of eosinophils, in a time- and dose-dependent fashion, at concentrations from 10^{-5} to 10^{-8} M, lyso-PAF had minimal activity over the same dose range (8). When PAF was compared with several other documented chemoattractants for eosinophil chemotaxis the rank order of potency (using optimal eosinophilotactic concentrations) was PAF $\geqslant$ C5a $>$ C5a$_{Des\ arg}$ = LTB$_4$ $>$ fMLP (14). In fact, compared with PAF, the eosinophil locomotory responses to LTB$_4$, histamine and the valyl and alanyl eosinophil tetrapeptides were negligible (8).

We recently established that PAF-induced eosinophil locomotion can be inhibited by a specific PAF antagonist derived from *Gingko biloba* (BN 52021) (16). In response to an optimal concentration of PAF (10^{-6} M) the drug was significantly more potent ($p < 0.001$) in inhibiting eosinophil as compared with neutrophil locomotion (Fig. 1). These inhibitory effects were observed in a dose-dependent manner with an IC$_{50}$ of 7.0 ($\pm$ 2.2) $\times$ 10^{-6} M and 2.3 ($\pm$ 0.2) $\times$ 10^{-5} M, for eosinophils and neutrophils, respectively. Sodium cromoglycate, nedocromil sodium, salbutamol and dexamethasone (pre-incubated with cells for up to 6 h) had no effect. Inhibition by BN 52021 was specific for PAF, in that it had no effect on chemotaxis induced by either LTB$_4$, *N*-formyl-methionyl-leucyl-phenylalanine (fMLP) or a purified human mononuclear cell-derived neutrophil chemotactic factor. BN 52021 also inhibited the specific binding of [^{3}H]-PAF (10^{-8} M) to eosinophils and neutrophils, in a concentration-dependent fashion. These results suggest that BN 52021 has potential as an anti-inflammatory agent in conditions associated with PAF-induced accumulation of neutrophils and eosinophils.

15.3   PAF AND EOSINOPHIL MEMBRANE RECEPTORS

Activation of eosinophils by PAF has been studied in a variety of systems. For instance, PAF (at an optimal concentration of 10^{-7} M) gave dose- and

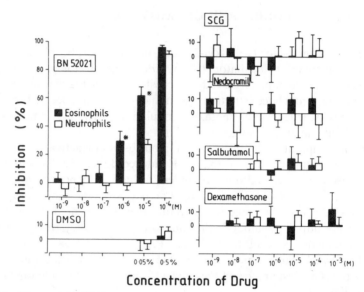

Concentration of Drug

Fig. 1 Effects of BN 52021, sodium cromoglycate, nedocromil sodium, salbutamol and dexamethasone on PAF-induced (10^{-6} M) eosinophil (closed bar) and neutrophil (open bar) chemotaxis. Drugs were added to both upper and lower chemotaxis chambers at the beginning of the chemotaxis assay. Diluent of BN 52021, HBSS or RMPI containing equivalent concentrations of DMSO, did not influence the chemotaxis significantly. Each point represents the mean ± SEM of 3 to 10 experiments. * significant ($p < 0.001$) differences between the inhibition of eosinophil and neutrophil chemotaxis. (Reproduced from ref. 16.)

time-dependent increases in the expression of membrane receptors as measured by IgE, IgG and complement rosettes on normal density eosinophils (17). At 10^{-5} M histamine also produced a small, but significant, percentage enhancement of eosinophil IgE and IgG rosettes. In contrast, fMLP (10^{-8} M) enhanced IgG-, but not IgE-dependent, rosettes. In all instances, rosette enhancement was maximal at 30 min after incubation with the activating agent, although still significantly above baseline at 60 min. These findings were extended using flow cytometry (since rosetting is essentially a semi-quantitative technique, unable to identify subtle changes in receptor expression and may be influenced by other non-specific membrane ligands). BB10, the monoclonal antibody described as recognising FcεRII on some hypodense eosinophils, gives very weak fluorescence on low and normal density eosinophils in our hands as do other anti-CD23 monoclonal antibodies such as MHM6 and Mab25. FcεRII expression was therefore studied using an excess of native human myeloma IgE and a fluorescein-conjugated polyclonal anti-IgE to detect bound IgE (18).

Using this system we were able, in the first instance, to detect the presence of cytophilic IgE on resting normal density eosinophils (incubation with native myeloma IgE having no further effect on anti-IgE). This suggested that there was a subpopulation of normal density eosinophils which expressed FcεRII, most of which are occupied by cytophilic IgE. In this respect the findings of Capron et al. (5) were of interest since these investigations found that low density cells bound increased amounts of native IgE without stimulation in vitro. This was further evidence that such cells were "activated" compared with normal density eosinophils. We then showed that FcεRII could be upregulated since preincubation of eosinophils with PAF (10^{-7} M) gave a time- and dose-dependent increase in IgE binding. A smaller, but significant, difference was also observed with LTB_4 (10^{-7} M) and histamine (10^{-5} M). Lyso-PAF or diluent alone had no effect at any of the concentrations used. In time-course studies, PAF and LTB_4 gave significant increases in IgE binding after 5 min pre-incubation, with optimal effect at 30 min.

The complement receptors CR1 and CR3 were also studied on normal density eosinophils using monoclonal antibodies; CR1 is expressed in low numbers but CR3 is expressed in greater density and gives very bright fluorescence. When stimulated, normal density eosinophils showed enhanced expression of CR1 and CR3 in response to PAF but not lyso-PAF in a time- and concentration-dependent fashion similar to that of FcεRII. In Figure 2 up-regulation of CR3 on eosinophils and neutrophils by PAF is shown using two colour flow cytometry. Both cells express similar amounts of CR3 but cytofluorimetry allows eosinophils to be distinguished from neutrophils by their differential expression of Fcγ receptors. Neutrophils express FcγRII (CD32) and FcγRIII (CD16), while eosinophils only express FcγRII (Adele Hartnell, unpublished observations).

The effector function of eosinophils, as measured by their ability to adhere to and kill appropriately-opsonized helminthic targets in vitro, was also enhanced by prior stimulation of cells with PAF (17). Using preparations of IgG- and IgE-rich fractions of immune serum PAF (at an optimal dose of 10^{-8} M), but not lyso-PAF, produced 185%, 106% and 100% enhancement of eosinophil cytotoxicity against schistosomula of Schistosoma mansoni coated with IgE, IgG and complement, respectively. LTB_4 also enhanced killing by eosinophils of larvae coated with IgE (95%) and IgG (70%). In contrast, fMLP (optimal dose of 10^{-7} M), enhanced the IgG- (56%) but not IgE-dependent cytotoxicity. This was in contrast to histamine which enhanced the IgE- (77%) but not IgG-dependent in vitro killing, albeit at a higher concentration of 10^{-5} M (19). These studies, which have used a combination of quantitative (i.e. flow cytometry) and functional assays, indicate that various mediators of hypersensitivity can activate human eosinophils in vitro, via

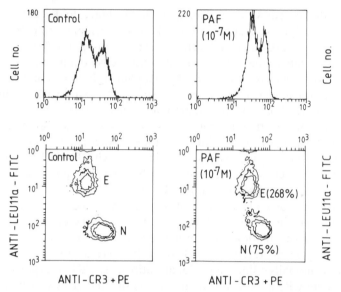

Fig. 2 Histograms of relative CR3 fluorescence (horizontal axis) against cell number (vertical axis) of a mixture of eosinophils and neutrophils incubated in either the absence (left), or presence of PAF (10^{-7} M) (right). The accompanying contour plots show the patterns of dual staining of the cell mixture (green fluorescence: vertical axis; red fluorescence: horizontal axis). Neutrophils stained with both monoclonal antibodies (anti-CR3 and anti-Leu 11b) whereas eosinophils staining only with anti-CR3. The enhancement of CR3 expression by PAF was 268% for eosinophils and 75% for neutrophils.

CR3 and FcεRII. PAF appears to be particularly effective in this respect and, since this agent has such a wide range of properties relevant to allergic inflammation, it may play a key role in IgE-related inflammatory responses both in allergy and acute immune reactions against helminthic parasites.

15.4   PAF AND LTC₄ GENERATION BY HUMAN EOSINOPHILS

PAF has been shown to be generated by several human cell types including macrophages, neutrophils, mast cells, and endothelial cells after a variety of physiologic and non-physiologic stimuli. PAF production by eosinophils, however, has been less well documented. One report describes activation of acetyl transferase and acetyl hydrolase (enzymes involved in PAF generation and breakdown respectively) by calcium ionophore and a variety of chemotactic factors (20). Generation of PAF itself was only briefly mentioned and restricted to the measurement of extra-cellular concentrations which were apparently very small (< 1 pg/10^6 cells).

We have previously shown that IgG-coated Sepharose beads are an effective stimulus for LTC_4 generation by eosinophils (7). We have therefore used the same stimulus to investigate PAF generation by normal and low density eosinophils and compared the results with those obtained with neutrophils. Neutrophils, normal density eosinophils and low density eosinophils generated PAF in a dose- and time-dependent manner in response to an IgG-coated bead stimulus (21). The greatest amounts of PAF were generated by normal density eosinophils. In all cell types most of the PAF generated was retained within the cells, although normal eosinophils released a greater proportion into the supernatant; fMLP also enhanced PAF generation by normal density eosinophils. Thus the eosinophil has the potential to generate physiologically active amounts of PAF and is therefore a likely source of this mediator in allergic inflammatory reactions.

As part of an ongoing study to identify a range of physiological triggers for LTC_4 production by eosinophils we have used specific immobilized IgG/antigen immune complexes to elicit mediator generation (22). An extract of *Aspergillus fumigatus* was covalently coupled to Sepharose beads and incubated with the IgG fraction of immune serum from patients with allergic bronchopulmonary aspergillosis (ABPA). These beads elicited generation of 7.72 ± 1.7 pmoles LTC_4 per 10^6 eosinophils as compared with 0.73 ± 0.19 pmoles/10^6 cells after eosinophils were incubated with beads treated with IgG from normal non-immune serum. The maximum antibody-dependent release achieved represented approximately 20% of that induced by the calcium ionophore (A23187). Grass pollen-specific IgG antibody/antigen complexes, in combination with Sepharose beads, also triggered generation of LTC_4 immunoreactive material.

An IgE myeloma protein, coupled to Sepharose beads, was a weak stimulus of LTC_4 generation by low-density cells. However, clearer evidence of IgE-dependent generation of LTC_4 from eosinophils was obtained using opsonized, formalin-fixed schistosomula (Sch) of *S. mansoni* (Table 1) (23). Sch were coated with either IgE or IgG fractions from immune serum separated by FPLC (Polyanion SI-17 column). IgE-rich fractions were identified by parasite-specific RAST and contaminating IgG removed by protein A adsorption. IgG-rich fractions were tested by specific ELISA and confirmed by adsorption on a *Staph. aureus* protein A affinity column. Low density eosinophils, incubated with live or fixed Sch coated with unfractionated immune serum released 16.5 ± 3.5 and 11.7 ± 2.7 pmoles of LTC_4/10^6 cells respectively. This compared with 80 ± 24 and 9.9 ± 1 pmoles in the presence of A23187 and IgG-coated beads, respectively. Fixed Sch coated with purified

Table 1   IgE- and IgG-mediated LTC$_4$ release from, and cytotoxicity of, low density human eosinophils

Opsonin	Specific anti-*schistosoma*		Hypodense eosinophils	
	IgG-ELISA (OD units)	IgE-RAST (% binding)	LTC$_4$ Release (pmoles/10^6 cells)	Cytotoxicity (% kill)
Unfractionated immune serum	8.4	36	15 ± 4	82 ± 5
IgG-rich fractions, untreated	6.8	0	6.0 ± 0.1	40 ± 2
IgG-rich fractions + Protein A	0.1	0	0.1 ± 0.1	9.4 ± 4
IgG-rich fractions + anti-IgE	6.0	0	5.6 ± 0.3	35 ± 3
IgE-rich fractions, untreated	7.0	35	7.8 ± 0.4	31 ± 1
IgE-rich fractions + Protein A	0.18	32	5.5 ± 0.4	30 ± 1.5
IgE-rich fractions + anti-IgE	6.4	0	0.25 ± 0.1	11 ± 2

Eosinophils were incubated with opsonised schistosomula of *S. mansoni* (formalin-fixed for LTC$_4$ release and live for killing assay). Larvae were coated with untreated immune (anti-*Schistosoma*) serum or FPLC-fractionated IgG- and IgE-rich pools. Parasite-specific IgG and IgE were measured by ELISA and RAST, respectively. IgG-depletion was achieved by adsorption on a protein A column; IgE was removed by an anti-IgE affinity column.

IgE and IgG fractions evoked the release of 7.6 ± 0.4 and 6.0 ± 0.1 pmoles of LTC$_4$ respectively per 10^6 low-density eosinophils. Adsorption of IgE on an anti-IgE column abolished the IgE-dependent release of LTC$_4$, while IgG-dependent generation was removed by protein A, but not anti-IgE adsorption. Thus the release of LTC$_4$ from eosinophils via IgE-dependent mechanisms following adherence to a helminth may aid in understanding the functional role of the FcεRII in allergy and immunity to helminths.

15.5   CLINICAL STUDIES ON EOSINOPHILS, ALLERGIC INFLAMMATION AND THE LATE-PHASE REACTION

Our group has also been concerned with attempts to provide direct evidence that eosinophils and their products play a role in tissue damage associated with allergic inflammation. One approach is to identify eosinophil granule products (as an index of activation) in tissues and body fluids and to relate such findings to clinical symptoms. An excellent model of allergen-induced inflammation is the late-phase reaction (LPR).

There have been a number of hypotheses which have sought to relate inflammatory cell infiltrates in LPRs to the subsequent clinical response. Early work suggested that immune complex deposition was important (24), but these claims have not been substantiated and, furthermore, the development or non-appearance of LPRs cannot be predicted from plasma levels of allergen-specific IgG, IgA and IgM. Indeed, allergen-specific IgG appears to attenuate the size of the cutaneous LPR rather than augment it (25). The ability of $F(ab')_2$ fractions of anti-IgE to elicit LPRs in normal human skin (26) suggested that the LPR was entirely mast cell-dependent, with cellular infiltration being secondary to the release of mast cell-derived chemotactic factors. However, the recognition that receptors for IgE (FcεRII) exist on macrophages (27), eosinophils (28), platelets (29) and T lymphocytes (30) suggests that other cell types may be involved in IgE-mediated reactions. Moreover, drugs such as salbutamol, which are effective mast cell stabilizers, do not prevent the development of the LPR (31). On the other hand, corticosteroids, which are extremely effective anti-inflammatory agents, do not influence the immediate allergic response (when given immediately prior to allergen challenge), but are very effective at blocking LPRs in the skin, nose and lung (32).

15.5.1   Eosinophils and Cutaneous Late-phase Reactions

Late-phase allergic reactions provoked either by specific allergen or by anti-IgE are associated with an intense inflammatory cell infiltrate consisting of eosinophils, neutrophils and mononuclear cells (26, 33, 34). In humans, late-phase reactions (i.e. the delay in time response observed 3–9 h after allergen administration) are seen in the lungs, nose, skin and conjunctiva. Although there has been a longstanding debate regarding the frequency of occurrence of the late-phase reaction, it now seems likely that LPRs can be elicited in all sensitized individuals and animals, provided enough allergen is administered. This view is based, first, on studies using intradermal injection of anti-IgE in non-atopic volunteers (26) and, secondly, on recent work in which we have shown that cutaneous LPRs could be elicited in all atopic subjects, provided sufficient allergen was injected (35). However, the magnitude of the late-phase skin reaction clearly varies considerably between individuals following weal and flare responses of similar size (26, 33, 35).

It has been appreciated for some time that in the late-phase skin reaction, in addition to eosinophils and neutrophils, there is a rich infiltration of mononuclear cells (33, 34). Since it is now clear that T cell products regulate the production and activation of eosinophils, it seemed reasonable to hypothesize that there may be an appreciable T cell component of the LPR, at least in the skin and that this, in turn, might be related to the intense eosinophilia.

Table 2   The numbers of infiltrating activated T lymphocytes and eosinophils in allergen-induced late-phase skin reactions

Mab	6 h	Mean Cells per Field 24 h	48 h	(Highest control)
CD3	17.42[b]	13.27[a]	10.98[b]	(5.69)
CD4	11.08[a]	11.45[b]	6.70[a]	(4.72)
IL-2R	0.18 NS	0.28[a]	0.39[a]	(0.10)
CD8	2.62 NS	2.03 NS	1.52 NS	(1.22)
EG2	14.82[c]	8.31[b]	7.90[b]	(0.64)

Mean number of positively stained cells per field in each group of subjects. Statistical comparisons by student's t test.
([a] $p < 0.05$, [b] $p < 0.01$, [c] $p < 0.0001$)

Late-phase skin reactions were induced in subjects with atopic rhinitis by intradermal injection of allergen extracts. Three groups of subjects were used, in whom biopsies were taken after 6, 24 and 48 h respectively. The groups were well matched for age and sex and the size of the weal and LPRs were comparable in all three groups. Six-micron thick cryostat sections were cut, fixed in acetone and methanol (50:50) and stained with monoclonal antibodies using the alkaline phosphatase anti-alkaline phosphatase (APAAP) technique. Numerous activated eosinophils were present at the site of allergen challenge, as indicated by staining with the monoclonal antibody EG2. These cells and their debris persisted for up to 48 h. T lymphocytes were also attracted to the cutaneous LPRs: substantial numbers were present by 6 h and T lymphocytes persisted for up to 48 h. The mean number of cells stained with each of the monoclonal antibodies is shown in Table 2. The majority of the infiltrating T lymphocytes were CD4 + and the infiltration appeared to be specific in that the CD4 +/CD8 + ratio of cells in the skin differed substantially from that measured in the blood. A small number of cells expressed the IL-2 receptor, providing evidence of T cell activation. Supporting this observation, there was increased expression of HLA-DR by endothelial cells and of CD4 antigen by epidermal Langerhans cells, changes which are thought to be mediated by the T cell product, interferon-γ (36, 37).

Linear regression analysis showed a correlation between the diameter of the LPR (measured at 6 h) and the number of activated eosinophils at 48 h ($r = 0.61$, $p = 0.05$). There was no clear association of LPR size with any of the T cell subsets but there was a strong association between the number of CD4 + T cells and the number of activated eosinophils at 24 h ($r = 0.94$, $p < 0.001$) with a similar, but statistically non-significant trend at 48 h ($r = 0.54$). These findings suggest that CD4 + T lymphocytes and their products, together with eosinophils and their mediators contribute to the pathogenesis of chronic allergic inflammation.

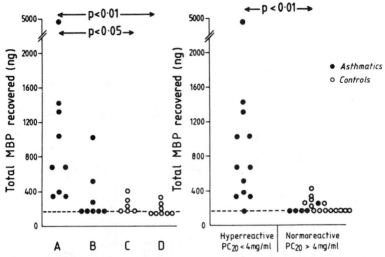

Fig. 3   Amount of MBP (ng) recovered from the BAL in four groups of subjects (A, symptomatic asthmatics; B, asymptomatic asthmatics; C, hayfever sufferers; D, non-atopic normal controls) and comparison between hyperreactive and normoreactive subjects. The dotted lines represent amounts below the sensitivity of the assay. (Reproduced from ref. 38.)

There are several important issues raised by these experiments in terms of the expression of allergic responses. First, there is the question whether activated T lymphocytes play a role in ongoing chronic allergic diseases (including extrinsic asthma); secondly, there is the possibility that T lymphocytes play a part in recruiting granulocytes to sites of allergic inflammation; and, finally, there is the possibility that granulocytes, once recruited, may be activated locally by lymphokines and thereby acquire increased inflammatory potential.

15.5.2   Eosinophils and Late-phase Asthmatic Reactions

In symptomatic allergic asthmatics the numbers of eosinophils in bronchoalveolar lavage (BAL) (in the baseline, "resting" state) was significantly higher than in asymptomatic asthmatics, hay fever sufferers and normal nonatopic individuals (38). Similar increases were found in the concentrations of the eosinophil major basic protein (MBP), a major secretory product of activated eosinophils (Fig. 3). Furthermore, there were significant correlations between MBP concentrations and: (1) the degree of non-specific hyperresponsiveness; (2) the number of shed epithelial cells in BAL; and (3) the BAL eosinophil counts. These findings support the hypothesis that activated

BAL after allergen challenge in asthma

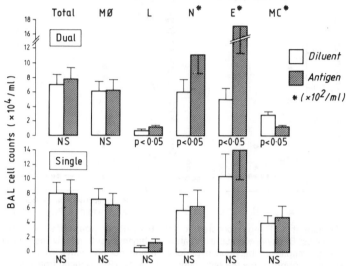

Fig. 4   Leucocyte and mast cell counts in BAL after diluent and antigen challenge in subjects with either dual reactions or single early reactions 6 h following antigen or diluent provocation. The data represent the means and standard errors ($n = 7$). Statistically significant differences "within groups" (Wilcoxon matched-pair test) are shown. "Between group" differences (Mann–Whitney U test) were not significant (NS).

eosinophils release MBP (and presumably other basic proteins from the crystalloid granule) which destroys epithelial cells and, in turn, accentuates bronchial hyperreactivity.

BAL studies of the human late asthmatic reaction have also revealed the presence of significantly increased numbers of eosinophils during the late response, whereas relatively modest increases were seen in single early responders (39). In a recent study we measured the total and differential cells counts, histamine, LTB_4 and LTC_4, immunoglobulins, complement (C), eosinophil-derived basic proteins, and monocyte complement rosettes (MCR) in BAL 6 h after challenge with either antigen (Ag) or diluent (D) control in 7 patients with antigen-induced single early reactions (SER), and 7 with dual (early- and late-phase) responses (43). In both groups the total cell counts in BAL were similar, irrespective of whether they were challenged with Ag or D. However, in LPR there were significant increases in lymphocytes, neutrophils and eosinophils, and significant decreases in the percentage of lung mast cells (Fig. 4). MBP and eosinophil-derived neurotoxin (EDN) increased in 4 out of 5 subjects with dual responses and most of the patients with SER. BAL histamine concentrations increased in 5 out of 7 patients with dual responses.

There were no consistent changes in LTB_4 concentrations in either the LPR or SER groups between diluent and antigen days, but a small but significant increase in LTC_4 was observed in the LPR group. Concentrations of IgG, IgA, IgM, IgE, C3 and albumin did not differ significantly. The percentage of monocyte complement rosettes also increased significantly ($p < 0.05$) in LPR, but not in SER. These findings support the hypothesis that eosinophils and their products play a role in tissue injury in LPR and that eosinophil infiltration may be associated with macrophage activation.

Our recent work also supports the hypothesis that T cell subsets may be involved in the expression of the late-phase asthmatic reaction in humans. Relative increases in CD8+ cells in BAL were seen in single early responders, as compared with late-phase responders (40). One other study has addressed this area, using segmental bronchial challenge via the fibre-optic broncho-scope in late responders, and demonstrated a selective increase in CD4+ cells in lavage fluid 48 h after challenge (41). These findings are also consistent with the reported decrease in CD4+ cells in the peripheral blood following allergen inhalation (42) and suggest a selective recruitment and retention of CD4+ T lymphocytes in the lungs during the late asthmatic reaction.

15.6   SUMMARY

Our studies indicate that human eosinophils can be activated in terms of up-regulation of surface receptors, increased membrane lipid generation and enhanced cytotoxicity, by a variety of pharmacological mediators through IgE-, IgG- and complement-dependent pathways. PAF is an impressive activator of eosinophil function and is the most potent chemotactic mediator for eosinophils so far described. It is not selective in that neutrophils are also attracted by PAF. In our hands, IL-1, IL-2, GM-CSF, TNF, IFN_γ and IL-5 tested over a wide concentration range gave very weak chemotaxis for eosinophils *in vitro*. Nevertheless, *in vivo* infiltration of eosinophils into the site of allergic tissue reactions is closely associated with the local accumulation of activated (CD4+, IL-2 rec+) T cells. Thus we suggest therefore that the selective eosinophil infiltration which is seen in allergic inflammation may result from the initial recruitment and activation of granulocytes by lipid mediators, and the subsequent selective activation of eosinophils by cytokines.

Acknowledgements

We are indebted to a number of our colleagues, both in the UK and abroad, who have contributed in many ways to the material presented here. In particular we wish to acknowledge Drs John Collins, Gerry Gleich, Pierre Braquet, Stephen Durham, Robyn O'Hehir, Piero Maestrelli, Rory Shaw, Mr Angus MacDonald and Miss Dawn Shepherd. This work was supported by the Wellcome Trust (UK), the Medical Research Council (UK), and the Clinical Research Committee of the National Heart and Chest Hospitals, London.

REFERENCES

1. Bass, D. A., Grover, W. H., Lewis, J. Szejda, P., De Chatelet, L. R. and McCall, C. E. (1980). Comparison of human eosinophils from normals and patients with eosinophilia. *J. Clin. Invest.* **66**, 1558–1564.
2. De Simone, D., Donelli, G., Mell, D., Rosati, F. and Sorice, F. (1982). Human eosinophils and parasitic diseases. II. Characterization of two cell fractions isolated at different densities. *Clin. Exp. Immunol.* **48**, 249–255.
3. Winqvist, I., Olofsson, T., Olsson, I., Persson, A-M. and Hallberg, T. (1982). Altered density, metabolism and surface receptors of eosinophils in eosinophilia. *Immunology* **47**, 531–539.
4. Prin, L., Charon, J., Capron, M., Gosset, P., Taelman, H., Tonnel, A. B. and Capron, A. (1984). Heterogeneity of human eosinophils. II. Variability of respiratory burst activity related to cell density. *Clin. Exp. Immunol.* **57**, 735–742.
5. Capron, M., Kusnierz, J. P. Prin, L. Spiegelberg, H. L., Ovlaque, G., Gosset, P., Tonnel, A. B. and Capron, A. (1985). Cytophilic IgE on human blood and tissue eosinophils: detection of flow microfluorometry. *J. Immunol.* **134**, 3013–3018.
6. Capron, M., Spiegelberg, H. L., Prin, L., Bennich, H., Butterworth, A. E., Pierce, R. J., Aliouaissi, M. and Capron, M. (1984). Role of IgE receptors in effector function of human eosinophils. *J. Immunol.* **132**, 462–468.
7. Shaw, R. J., Walsh, G. M., Cromwell, O., Moqbel, R., Spry, C. J. F. and Kay, A. B. (1985). Activated human eosinophils generate SRS-A leukotrienes following physiological (IgG-dependent) stimulation. *Nature* **316**, 150–152.
8. Wardlaw, A. J., Moqbel, R., Cromwell, O. and Kay, A. B. (1986). Platelet activating factor. A potent chemotactic and chemokinetic factor for human eosinophils. *J. Clin. Invest.* **78**, 1701–1706.
9. Tai, P.-C. and Spry, C. J. F. (1976). Studies on blood eosinophils. I. Patients with a transient eosinophilia. *Clin. Exp. Immunol.* **24**, 415–422.
10. Tai, P.-C., Spry, C. J. F., Peterson, C., Venge, P. and Olsson, I. (1984). Monoclonal antibodies distinguish between storage and secreted forms of eosinophil cationic protein. *Nature* **309**, 182–184.
11. Silberstein, D. S., David, J. R. (1987). The regulation of human eosinophil function by cytokines. *Immunol. Today* **8**, 380–385.
12. Lopez, A. F., Sanderson, C. J., Gamble, J. R., Campbell, H. D., Young, I. G. and Vadas, M.A. (1988). Recombinant human interleukin 5 in a selective activator of human eosinophil function. *J. Exp. Med.* **167**, 219–224.

13. Yamaguchi, Y., Hayashi, Y., Sugama, Y., Miura, Y., Kasahara, T., Kitamura, S., Torisu, M., Mita, S., Tominaga, A., Takatsu, K. and Suda T. (1988). Highly purified murine interleukin 5 (IL-5) stimulates eosinophil function and prolongs *in vitro* survival. IL-5 is an eosinophil chemotactic factor. *J. Exp. Med.* **167**, 1737–1742.

14. Kurihara, K., Wardlaw, A. J., Maestrelli, P., Tsai, J.-J. and Kay, A. B. (1988). IL-1, IL-2, TNF, INF-γ, GM-CSF and PHA-stimulated leukocyte supernatants have negligible eosinophil chemotactic activity compared with platelet activating factor (PAF). *FASEB J.* **2**, A1449 (abstr. 6695).

15. Braquet, P., Touqui, L., Shen, T. Y. and Vargaftig, B. B. (1987). Prospectives in platelet activating factor research. *Pharmacol. Rev.* **39**, 97–145.

16. Kurihara, K., Wardlaw, A. J., Moqbel, R. and Kay, A. B. (1989). Inhibition of platelet activating factor (PAF)-induced chemotaxis, and PAF binding to human eosinophils and neutrophils by the specific gingkolide-derived PAF antagonist, BN 52021. *J. Allergy Clin. Immunol.* **83**, 83–90.

17. Moqbel, R., Walsh, G. M. MacDonald, A. J., Wardlaw, A. J. and Kay, A. B. (1987). Activation of human eosinophils by PAF-acether and other inflammatory mediators. *Thorax* **42**, 221 (abstr.).

18. Walsh, G. M., Nagakura, T., Moqbel, R., Kay, A. B. and Iikura, Y. (1989). Flow cytometric analysis of PAF-induced enhancement of eosinophil IgE binding. *Clin. Exp. Allergy* **19**, 107 (Abstract 85/9).

19. Moqbel, R., Walsh, G. M., MacDonald, A. J., Hartnell, A., Wardlaw, A. J., Kay, A. B. Activation of human eosinophils by the platelet activating factor and leukotriene B₄. (Submitted)

20. Lee, T. C., Lenihan, D. J., Malone, B., Ruddy, L.L. and Wasserman, S. I. (1984). Increased biosynthesis of platelet-activating factor in activated human eosinophils. *J. Biol. Chem.* **259**, 5526–5530.

21. Champion, A., Wardlaw, A. J., Moqbel, R., Cromwell, O., Shepherd, D. and Kay, A. B. (1988). IgG-dependent generation of platelet-activating factor by normal and 'low-density' human eosinophils. *J. Allergy Clin. Immunol.* **81**, 207 (abstr.).

22. Cromwell, O., Moqbel, R., Fitzharris, P., Kurlak, L., Harvey, C., Walsh, G. M., Shaw, R. J. and Kay, A. B. (1989). Leukotriene C₄ generation from human eosinophils stimulated with IgG-*Aspergillus fumigatus* antigen immune complexes. *J. Allergy Clin. Immunol.* **82**, 535–544.

23. Moqbel, R., MacDonald, A. J., Kay, A. B. (1988). IgE-dependent release of leukotriene (LT) C₄ from human low-density eosinophils. *J. Allergy Clin. Immunol.* **81**, 208 (abstr. 158).

24. Pepys, J., Turner-Warwick, M., Dawson, P. and Hinson, K. F. W. (1968). Arthus (type III) skin test reactions in man. Clinical and immunopathological features. *In* "Allergology" (Eds B. Rose, R. Richter, S. Sehon and A. W. Frankland) 221–235. *Int. Congr. Ser.* **162**. Excerpta Med, Amsterdam.

25. Zetterstrom, O. (1978). Dual skin test reactions and serum antibodies to subtilisin and Aspergillus fumigatus extracts. *Clin. Allergy* **8**, 77–87.

26. Dolovich, J., Hargreave, F. E., Chalmers, R., Shier, K. J., Gauldie, J. and Bienenstock, J. (1973). Late cutaneous allergic responses in isolated IgE-dependent reactions. *J. Allergy Clin. Immunol.* **52**, 38–46.

27. Melewicz, F. M. and Spiegelberg, H. L. (1980). Fc receptors for IgE on a subpopulation of human peripheral blood monocytes. *J. Immunol.* **125**, 1026–1031.

28. Capron, M., Capron, A., Dessaint, J.-P., Torpier, G., Johansson, S. G. O. and

Prin. L. (1981). Fc receptors for IgE on human and rat eosinophils. *J. Immunol.* **126**, 2087–2092.

29. Joseph, M., Capron, A., Ameisen, J. C., Capron, M., Vorng, H., Pancré, V., Kusnierz, J. P. and Auriault, C. (1986). The receptor for IgE on blood platelets. *Eur. J. Immunol.* **16**, 306–312.

30. Prinz, J. C., Baur, X., Ring, J., Endres, N. and Rieker, E. P. (1988). Allergen induced Fc receptors for IgE on human T lymphocytes. *J. Allergy Clin. Immunol.* **81**, 304.

31. Twentyman, O. P. and Holgate, S. T. (1987). Pharmacological modification of the late asthmatic response and effects on circulating inflammatory cells. *J. Allergy Clin. Immunol.* **79**, 150.

32. Booij-Noord, H., Orie, N. G. and DeVries, K. (1971). Immediate and late bronchial obstructive reactions to inhalation of house dust and protective effects of disodium cromoglycate and prednisolone. *J. Allergy Clin. Immunol.* **48**, 344–354.

33. Solley, G., Gleich, G. J. Jordan, R. and Schroeter, A. L. (1976). The late phase of the immediate wheal and flare skin reactions: its dependence upon IgE antibodies. *J. Clin. Invest.* **58**, 408–420.

34. Richerson, H. B., Rajtora, D., Penick, G., Dick, F. R., Yoo, T. J., Kammermeyer, J. K. and Anuras, J. S. (1979). Cutaneous and nasal allergic responses in ragweed hay fever: lack of clinical and histopathological correlation with late phase reactions. *J. Allergy Clin. Immunol.* **64**, 67–77.

35. Frew, A. J. and Kay, A. B. (1989). The pattern of late phase allergic skin reactions in man. *J. Allergy Clin. Immunol.* **81**, 1117–1121.

36. Bevilacqua, M. P., Pober, J. S., Majeau, G. R., Cotran, R. S. and Gimbrone, M.A. Jr. (1984). Interleukin 1 induces biosynthesis and cell surface expression of procoagulant activity in human vascular endothelial cells. *J. Exp. Med.* **160**, 618–623.

37. Walsh, L. J., Parry, A., Scholes, A. and Seymour, G. J. (1987). Modulation of CD4 antigen on human gingival Langerhans cells by gamma interferon. *Clin. Exp. Immunol.* **70**, 379–382.

38. Wardlaw, A. J., Dunnette, S., Gleich, G. J., Collins, J. V. and Kay, A. B. (1988). Eosinophils and mast cells in bronchoalveolar lavage in mild asthma: relationship to bronchial hyperreactivity. *Am. Rev. Respir. Dis.* **137**, 62–69.

39. De Monchy, J. G. R., Kauffman, H. F., Venge, P., Koeter, G. H., Jansen, H. M., Sleuter, H. J. and DeVries, K. (1985). Bronchoalveolar eosinophilia during allergen-induced late asthmatic reactions. *Am. Rev. Respir. Dis.* **131**, 373–376.

40. Gonzalez, M. C., Diaz, P., Galleguillos, F. R., Ancic, P., Cromwell, O. and Kay, A. B. (1987). Allergen-induced recruitment of bronchoalveolar (OKT4) and suppressor (OKT8) cells in asthma. Relative increases on OKT8 cells in single early responders compared with those in late-phase responders. *Am. Rev. Respir. Dis.* **136**, 600–604.

41. Metzger, W. J., Zavala, D., Richerson, H. B., Moseley, P., Iwamota, P., Monick, M., Sjoerdsma, K. and Hunninghake, G. W. (1987). Local allergen challenge and bronchoalveolar lavage of allergic asthmatic lungs. Description of the model and local airway inflammation. *Am. Rev. Respir. Dis.* **135**, 433–440.

42. Gerblich, A. A., Campbell, A. and Schuyler, M. (1984). Changes in T lymphocyte subpopulations after antigenic bronchial provocation in asthmatics. *N. Engl. J. Med.* **310**, 1349–1352.

43. Diaz, P. *et al.* (1989). Leukocytes and mediators in bronchoalveolar lavage during late-phase asthmatic reactions. *Am. Rev. Respir. Dis.* (in press).

16

The Eosinophil and Asthma

G. J. Gleich

Department of Immunology and Internal Medicine,
Division of Allergic Diseases,
Mayo Clinic and Mayo Foundation, Mayo Medical School, Rochester, MN 55905, USA

16.1 INTRODUCTION

Soon after Ehrlich discovered the eosinophil leukocyte in 1879 (1), Ellis described the association of blood and tissue eosinophilia with asthma (2). In 1922, Huber and Koessler highlighted the massive blood and tissue eosinophilia in the lungs of patients dying of asthma (3). In the 1930s Kallos and Pagel first noted bronchial eosinophilia of sensitive guinea-pigs nebulized with antigen and called attention to the similarity to fatal cases of human asthma (4). In 1975, Horn and colleagues demonstrated that, in patients with asthma, the greater the number of eosinophils in the peripheral blood, the lower the FEV_1 (5). The simplest hypothesis for the observations of Horn *et al.* is that the eosinophil contributes directly to the pathophysiological processes responsible for bronchial asthma. By the late 1970s, a considerable body of evidence had accumulated that eosinophils kill helminths (6, 7), and

Eosinophils in Asthma
ISBN 0-12-506452-7

mammalian cells (8), through an antibody-dependent cell-mediated cytotoxicity. These findings raised the possibility that the same toxic properties of the eosinophil which are beneficial when focused on an invading helminth might be turned against the host in diseases characterized by prominent tissue eosinophilia such as bronchial asthma.

Information supporting the hypothesis that the eosinophil is a mediator of the pathophysiology of bronchial asthma was reviewed in detail (9). Here the eosinophil hypothesis will be examined in the light of recent findings showing that several eosinophil granule proteins are toxic to respiratory epithelium and that eosinophil degranulation occurs in damaged epithelium both in the upper and lower airways. Finally, the possibility that the eosinophil mediates damage to respiratory epithelium and, thus, underlies bronchial hyperreactivity will be discussed.

16.2   EOSINOPHILS AND TISSUE DAMAGE IN ASTHMA

Prior studies had established that MBP (10–12) was toxic to guinea-pig and human respiratory epithelium (13–15). In the present experiments, the ability of other eosinophil granule proteins, including eosinophil cationic protein (ECP), eosinophil-derived neurotoxin (EDN) and eosinophil peroxidase (EPO) (reviewed in 16), to cause damage to guinea pig tracheal epithelium in vitro was tested (17). Examination by inverted microscopy revealed that MBP, ECP and EPH + H_2O_2 + halide, but not EDN, caused dose-related damage to the tracheal epithelium. The lowest concentrations of MBP and ECP causing damage were 10 μg/ml and 100 μg/ml, respectively. In contrast, EDN, although biochemically similar to ECP, did not damage the tracheal epithelium up to 200 μg/ml. EPO in the presence of the H_2O_2-producing enzyme glucose oxidase (GO), Cl^-, 0.11 M, and iodide (10^{-4} M) caused ciliostasis, bleb formation, and exfoliation of epithelial cells at concentrations as low as 1–10 μg/ml. EPO + GO in the presence of Cl^-, 0.11 M, alone or with Cl^- and I^-, 10^{-4} M or Cl^- and Br^-, 5×10^{-5} M, were all toxic to epithelium. Surprisingly, EPO by itself caused ciliostasis, bleb formation and exfoliation of epithelial cells at concentrations as low as 1 U/ml (4.1 μg/ml). These results confirm prior observations on the toxicity of MBP to tracheal epithelium and indicate that ECP and EPO alone, as well as EPO + GO + halide, cause damage. Thus, several eosinophil granule proteins are able to damage respiratory epithelium.

Prior studies of MBP had also shown that ciliated cells are damaged, as judged by reduction or frank cessation, in the beating of the cilia (13–15). In recent experiments, selected regions of the epithelial surface of rabbit tracheal explants were videotaped before and after treatment with human MBP to quantify ciliary damage (18). Tapes were analysed for ciliary beat frequency and the extent of zones along the epithelial surface displaying ciliary activity. MBP at 100 and 700 μg/ml reduced both beat frequency and the measured zones of ciliary activity. Beat frequency was lowered by 27% within 10 min, and only decreased 1% further by 60 min. The zones of ciliary activity on the epithelium were continuously decreased throughout the 60 min to 29% of the zone initially active. To examine whether human MBP was capable of direct inhibition of ciliary activity, isolated porcine tracheal ciliary axonemes, the structural organelles of individual cilia, were treated with MBP. MBP concentrations above 67 μg/ml of human MBP were completely inhibitory to reactivated isolated axonemes, MBP, 67 μg/ml, stopped activity within 10 min, and MBP, 27 μg/ml, stopped activity within 15 min. Pretreatment of isolated axonemes with increasing concentrations of human MBP resulted in decreasing ATPase activity. These effects were not attributable to pH change. No changes in axonemal protein bands were observed in sodium dodecyl sulphate-polyacrylamide gradient gel electrophoresis, except for the presence of MBP in axonemal samples treated with MBP. These results suggested that MBP can inhibit the activity of ciliated cells and can directly impair axonemal function probably by inhibition of ATPase activity. The significance of these observations rests on the likelihood that these reactions occur *in vivo* during asthma. Levels of MBP up to 93 μg/ml (7×10^{-6} M) have been measured in sputum (15) of patients with asthma, and MBP has been localized to sites of damage on bronchial epithelium (19). Although the local concentrations of MBP in damaged tissues are not known, they are probably in excess of 1×10^{-5} M. Thus, the concentrations of MBP employed in these studies may be achieved *in vivo* at sites of eosinophil degranulation and may contribute to epithelial damage. The subsequent inadequate ciliary clearance would prolong exposure to MBP and other potentially injurious compounds such as EPO and ECP, extending tissue destruction.

16.3   DEPOSITION OF MBP ON DAMAGED RESPIRATORY EPITHELIUM

The information summarized above indicates that MBP, EPO and ECP have the potential to cause damage to respiratory epithelium. This hypothesis has been supported by the finding in tissue specimens of patients dying of asthma and in tissues from paranasal sinuses that MBP is deposited at sites of damaged epithelium (19–21). In the initial studies of the localization of MBP in bronchial asthma, MBP deposition outside the eosinophil was observed: (1) in mucus plugs; (2) in the submucosa in association with apparent eosinophil degranulation; and (3) on the surface of denuded bronchial epithelium (19). However, in these studies there was no evidence of MBP deposition on to epithelium which was in the process of desquamation. Re-investigation of cases of fatal asthma (20) has employed specimens from the cases reported by Kravis and Kolski (22). These autopsy specimens have shown striking eosinophil degranulation at the bases of denuded areas of epithelium and, in some cases, frank disruption of the basement membrane zone. In other areas, MBP was deposited on to apparently desquamated clumps of epithelial cells in the lumen of the bronchiole. These clumps likely correspond to Creola bodies (23, 24). MBP can also be seen coating the surface of the epithelium in the absence of obvious cell damage; as indicated below, such MBP deposition could still alter the functioning of the epithelium.

In collaboration with Harlin and his associates, we have studied paranasal sinus tissue from patients with asthma and/or allergic rhinitis obtained at the time of performance of Caldwell–Luc procedures (21). Localization of MBP by immunofluorescence showed a spectrum of changes ranging from intact epithelium and an absence of eosinophils to complete loss of epithelium and marked eosinophilia and eosinophil degranulation. Areas of epithelium undergoing marked desquamation showed intense extracellular fluorescent staining for MBP, indicating that extensive eosinophil degranulation had occurred. At the opposite end of the spectrum, where sinus epithelium was intact, a paucity of eosinophils was observed with minimal or no extracellular MBP deposition. Taken together, these findings are in accord with the hypothesis that MBP damages paranasal respiratory epithelium in a manner similar to that described in chronic asthma.

16.4   A MECHANISM FOR THE INDUCTION OF BRONCHIAL HYPERREACTIVITY IN ASTHMA

The information summarized above supports the hypothesis that the eosinophil through its complement of toxic granule proteins causes damage to and desquamation of bronchial epithelial cells. Dysfunction or loss of respiratory epithelial cells may contribute to the bronchial hyperreactivity associated with asthma (25–27). Loss of epithelial cells alters the osmolarity of the mucosal surface (26) and exposes underlying sensory nerves (25), possibly leading to bronchoconstriction. Epithelial cells could also release a relaxing

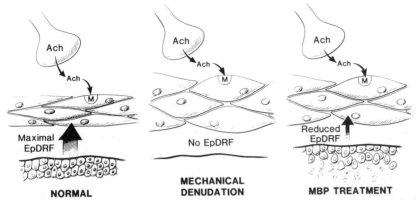

Fig. 1 Schematic diagram of the relationships between the effects of epithelial-derived relaxing factor (EpDRF) and acetylcholine (Ach) on respiratory smooth muscle. M denotes the muscarinic receptor and MBP denotes the eosinophil granule major basic protein. In the presence of normal epithelium and maximal levels of EpDRF, smooth muscle is relatively relaxed (left). After mechanical denudation of epithelium, EpDRF is absent and smooth muscle is contracted due to the unbalanced effect of Ach. After MBP treatment, EpDRF is reduced and smooth muscle is relatively contracted.

factor(s) causing relaxation of the underlying smooth muscle. Removal of the epithelium from canine bronchi *in vitro* increases the sensitivity of the bronchial smooth muscle to several agonists, including acetylcholine, 5-hydroxytryptamine and histamine, but reduces the relaxant potency of isoproterenol (28). The putative epithelium-derived relaxing factor(s) can be detected in bioassay experiments (29, 30). By interfering with the release of this relaxing factor, damage to the epithelial cells may cause hyperreactivity of bronchial smooth muscle, as occurs *in vitro* (28, 29, 31–33).

We have recently analysed whether MBP (100 μg/ml) can directly influence the reactivity of respiratory smooth muscle *in vitro* (34). The sensitivity to histamine and acetylcholine of rings of guinea-pig trachea, some with and some without epithelium, was determined under control conditions and following incubation with MBP (100 μg/ml). MBP did not affect the contractile activity of rings of guinea-pig trachea which had previously been denuded of epithelium, indicating that the protein at this concentration is not cytotoxic toward smooth muscle cells. However, when MBP was incubated with tracheal preparations having an intact epithelial cell layer, MBP caused augmentation of the contractile responses to acetylcholine and histamine. The most likely explanation is that MBP, by damaging the epithelial cells, had inhibited the release of some, as yet unidentified, epithelium-derived relaxing factor(s). Although the functional studies suggest that MBP has interfered with epithelial cell function, light microscopy revealed that MBP (100 μg/ml) did not cause epithelial desquamation. The results therefore suggest that MBP, in concentrations which do not cause frank epithelial denudation, can either interfere sufficiently with epithelial cell function to cause interruption of the release of epithelium-derived relaxing factor(s) or that MBP interferes with the diffusion and/or action of the released factor(s) (Fig. 1). An alternative explanation is that MBP changes the metabolism of the epithelial cells from the production of smooth muscle relaxant factors to the generation of constrictor factors.

Degranulation of eosinophils and the subsequent deposition of toxic proteins on to the surface of the epithelium may, therefore, contribute to the bronchial hyperreactivity that occurs in asthma by causing loss of or damage to epithelial surface. This in turn will result in a reduction of the activity of the epithelium-derived relaxing factor(s) thus causing hyperresponsiveness of the underlying smooth muscle. Although other factors (e.g. viral and bacterial infections) may contribute to epithelial dysfunction, and this dysfunction may also affect smooth muscle responsiveness, this model provides a basis for the hyperreactivity associated with the chronic inflammation seen in asthma.

Acknowledgements

Supported by grants from the National Institutes of Health, AI 09728, AI 15231, and AI 11483, and from the Mayo Foundation.

REFERENCES

1. Ehrlich, P. (1879). Bietrage zur Kenntnis der granulirten Bindegewebszellen und der eosinophilen leukocythen. *Arch. Anat. Physiol. (Physiol. Abt.)* **166**.
2. Ellis, A. G. (1908). The pathological anatomy of bronchial asthma. *Am. J. Med. Sci.* **136**, 407.
3. Huber, H. L. and Koessler, K. K. (1922). The pathology of bronchial asthma. *Arch. Intern. Med.* **30**, 689.
4. Kallos, P. and Kallos, L. (1984). Experimental asthma in guinea pigs revisited. *Int. Archs. Allergy appl. Immun.* **73**, 77.
5. Horn, B. R., Robin, E. D., Theodore, J. and Van Kessel, A. (1975). Total eosinophil counts in the management of bronchial asthma. *N. Engl. J. Med.* **292**, 1152.
6. Butterworth, A. E., Sturrock, R. F., Houba, V., Mahmoud, A. A. F., Sher, A. and Rees, P. H. (1975). Eosinophils as mediators of antibody-dependent damage to schistosomula. *Nature* **256**, 727.
7. Butterworth, A. E., Wassom, D. L., Gleich, G. J., Loegering, D. A. and David, J. R. (1979). Damage to schistosomula of *Schistosoma mansoni* induced directly by eosinophil major basic protein. *J. Immunol.* **122**, 221.

8. Parrillo, J. E., Fauci, A. S. (1978). Human eosinophils. Purification and cytotoxic capability of eosinophils from patients with the hypereosinophilic syndrome. *Blood* **51**, 457.
9. Frigas, E. and Gleich, G. J. (1986). The eosinophil and the pathophysiology of asthma. *J. Allergy Clin. Immunol.* **77**, 527.
10. Gleich, G. J., Loegering, D. A. and Maldonado, J. E. (1973). Identification of a major basic protein in guinea pig eosinophil granules. *J. Exp. Med.* **137**, 1459.
11. Gleich, G. J., Loegering, D. A., Kueppers, F., Bajaj, S. P. and Mann, K. G. (1974). Physiochemical and biological properties of the major basic protein from guinea pig eosinophil granules. *J. Exp. Med.* **140**, 313.
12. Gleich, G. J., Loegering, D. A., Mann, K. G. and Maldonado, J. E. (1976). Comparative properties of the Charcot-Leyden crystal protein and the major basic protein from human eosinophils. *J. Clin. Invest.* **57**, 633.
13. Gleich, G. J., Frigas, E., Loegering, D. A., Wassom, D. L. and Steinmuller, D. (1979). Cytotoxic properties of the eosinophil major basic protein. *J. Immunol.* **123**, 2925.
14. Frigas, E., Loegering, D. A. and Gleich, G. J. (1980). Cytotoxic effects of the guinea pig eosinophil major basic protein on tracheal epithelium. *Lab. Invest.* **42**, 35.
15. Frigas, E., Loegering, D. A., Solley, G. O., Farrow, G. M. and Gleich, G. J. (1981). Elevated levels of the eosinophil granule major basic protein in the sputum of patients with bronchial asthma. *Mayo Clin. Proc.* **56**, 345.
16. Gleich, G. J. and Adolphson, C. R. (1986). The eosinophilic leukocyte: structure and function. *Adv. Immunol.* **39**, 177.
17. Motojima, S., Loegering, D. A., Frigas, E. and Gleich, G. J. (1986). Toxic effects of eosinophil granule cationic proteins on respiratory epithelium. *Fed. Proc.* **45**, (Abst.), 994.
18. Hastie, A. T., Loegering, D. A., Gleich, G. J. and Kueppers, F. (1987). The effect of purified human eosinophil major basic protein on mammalian ciliary activity. *Am. Rev. Respir. Dis.* **135**, 848.
19. Filley, W. V., Holley, K. E., Kephart, G. M. and Gleich, G. J. (1982). Identification by immunofluorescence of eosinophil granule major basic protein in lung tissues of patients with bronchial asthma. *Lancet* **2**, 11.
20. Gleich, G. J., Motojima, S., Frigas, E., Kephart, G. M., Fujisawa, T. and Kravis, L. P. (1987). The eosinophilic leukocyte and the pathology of fatal bronchial asthma: Evidence for pathologic heterogeneity. *J. Allergy Clin. Immunol.* **80**, 412.
21. Harlin, S. L., Ansel, D. G., Lane, S. R., Myers, J., Kephart, G. M. and Gleich, G. J. (1988). A clinical and pathological study of chronic sinusitis: The role of the eosinophil. *J. Allergy Clin. Immunol.* **81**, 867.
22. Kravis, L. P. and Kolski, G. B. (1985). Unexpected death in childhood asthma: a review of 13 deaths in ambulatory patients. *Am. Dis. Child.* **139**, 558.
23. Naylor, B. (1962). The shedding of the mucosa of the bronchial tree in asthma. *Thorax* **17**, 69.
24. Naylor, B. (1985). Creola bodies: their discovery and significance. *Cytochem. Bull.* **22**, 33.
25. Nadel, J. A. (1983). Bronchial reactivity. *Adv. Intern. Med.* **28**, 207.
26. Hogg, J. C. and Eggleston, P. A. (1984). Is asthma an epithelial disease? *Am. Rev. Respir. Dis.* **129**, 207.
27. Laitinen, L. A., Heino, M., Laitinen, A., Kava, T. and Haahtela, T. (1985).

Damage of the airway epithelium and bronchial reactivity in patients with asthma. *Am. Rev. Respir. Dis.* **131**, 599.

28. Flavahan, N. A., Aarhus, L. L., Rimele, T. J. and Vanhoutte, P. M. (1985). Respiratory epithelium inhibits bronchial smooth muscle tone. *J. Appl. Physiol.* **58**, 834.
29. Vanhoutte, P. M. and Flavahan, N. A. (1988). Modulation of cholinergic neurotransmission in the airways. *In* "The Airways: Neural Control in Health and Disease" (Eds M. Kaliner and P. Barnes), 203–216. Dekker, New York.
30. Vanhoutte, P. M. (1987). Airway epithelium and bronchial reactivity. *Can. J. Physiol. Pharmacol.* **65**, 448.
31. Flavahan, N. A. and Vanhoutte, P. M. (1985). The respiratory epithelium releases a smooth muscle relaxing factor. *Chest* **87**, (Suppl.) 189.
32. Barnes, P. J., Cuss, F. M. and Palmer, J. B. (1985). The effect of airway epithelium on smooth muscle contractility in bovine trachea. *Br. J. Pharmacol.* **86**, 685.
33. Reaburn, D., Hay, D. W. P., Robinson, V. A., Farmer, S. G., Fleming, W. W. and Fedan, J. S. (1986). The effect of verapamil is reduced in isolated airway smooth muscle preparations lacking the epithelium. *Life Sci.* **38**, 809.
34. Flavahan, N. A., Slifman, N. R., Gleich, G. J. and Vanhoutte, P. M. (1988). Human eosinophil major basic protein causes hyperreactivity of respiratory smooth muscle. Role of the epithelium. *Am. Rev. Respir. Dis.* **138**, 685.

DISCUSSION

Dahl (Chairman): I wonder if, when you do chemotaxis studies with lavage fluid, donor cells from a normal person would differ from cells from an atopic person or the patient himself.

Kay: Yes, it is possible. We have very few chances with this rather precious material, so we opted to use normal normodense cells. But I agree, we might have got different results with more activated cells.

Gleich: Barry, what was the molecular weight of the major peak giving chemotactic activity?

Kay: 135 kilodaltons.

Gleich: I'm not aware of any eosinophil chemotactic factor at that molecular weight range.

Kay: Nor am I.

Wasserman: I don't know of any at that weight range, but you always have to worry about adherence of lower molecular weight materials to higher molecular weight carriers. One would want to do some kind of lipid extraction or salt extraction, to see what you had. I was curious, Barry—in your data, when you showed the elevated MBP levels in the bronchoalveolar lavage, how do you prevent the eosinophils that are in the lavage from releasing MBP or do you try? Is the assay an MBP on fluid phase MBP or total extracted MBP from the lavage?

Kay: No, it's fluid phase MBP, the cells are immediately centrifuged gently and the cell free supernatants are stored and then transported.

Wasserman: My experience is that there is an awful lot of mucus in lavage fluid which is very hard to centrifuge down. I'm just wondering if MBP in these fluid phase reactions is sometimes a fancy eosinophil count. How can we really know what's in fluid and what is in cells? Do you have an idea about that Jerry?

Gleich: Well, I think that when you have a lot of eosinophils around, you often see more MBP but you can also see quite the opposite as well. You can see a lot of eosinophils and not much MBP. So I think that when you see MBP, you have a good indication that degranulation is occurring. One point I will make is that this was a super blind study. We have no idea of the identity of the samples Barry sent us.

Dahl: But I guess you filter your sample, to get rid of the mucus before you take the supernatant?

Kay: I have to say that with the British patients, there was very little mucus, it was a bit of a surprise. They were really very mild patients. But the samples in the other study I showed you were filtered through gauze.

Dahl: Per Venge, I know you have data on eosinophil chemotactic factors.

Venge: Yes, I have. And one of the eosinophil chemotactic activities we have identified in asthmatics, in this case in plasma, is actually exactly at the same molecular size as you show, that is 150 000. I have a question to Jerry and a comment. First I would like to know, what is one unit in milligrams of EPO?

Gleich: There are 256 units per milligram, so one unit is 4 μg.

Venge: Because I can confirm that EPO is very toxic by itself without having H_2O_2 present. We have seen that in a number of different cellular systems at very comparable concentrations.

Gleich: That's heartening.

Sanjar: I have a comment about the nature of EDRF. I think that it is pretty well known to be nitrous oxide now.

Gleich: Is that from bronchial epithelium or from endothelium?

Sanjar: From the endothelium but there is very little reason to believe they're different, although it has not been formally confirmed. And secondly, how did you do the *in vitro* experiments with MBP which because of its basic nature would stick to the glass and tissues and other things?

Gleich: I have to confess we had to bubble oxygen through the solutions which got a little bit murky. When MBP was added to 100 μg it began to precipitate, as we know it does, so that actually the effective concentration was probably quite a bit lower. But in essence we simply took the native molecule at about 5 mg/ml off a column and added it in small quantities to achieve the concentration which was indicated.

Sanjar: Perhaps some of the effects you see are not specific to that molecule, but if you had another basic molecule, it may cause the same effect.

Gleich: In experiments which Dr Frigas did back in at about 1981 or '80, when protamine was put on respiratory epithelium, even though protamine is exceedingly basic with a molecular weight of 5000 kD and is almost all arginine, it caused relatively little damage, whereas in the same experiment MBP was causing lots of damage. So, I'm not absolutely certain that one could see comparable damage with another basic molecule. But having said that, I would quickly agree with you that basic proteins tend to be toxic. But on the other hand, this isn't just any basic protein, this is one in eosinophils which we associate with the pathology.

Dahl: Is there an effect of MBP on lymphocyte functions? I have read some data recently from Per Venge's laboratory which showed that MBP had influences on suppressor cells. Barry Kay showed us that OKT4 cells were decreased and OKT8 cells were increased after a challenge. Could this in some way be due to an effect of these basic proteins?

Gleich: Well, MBP is a powerful cytotoxin and will block the MLR, but if you leave it in there for very long, all the cells are dead, so the result is no surprise. We have, however, done titrations at quite low levels where one sees minimal if any toxicity and it also blocks the MLR. This information is intriguing to us because MBP is deposited in concentrations of the order of 10^{-5} M in the placenta at the fetal maternal interface deep to the chorionic villi and in fact extending into the myometrium.

Dahl: I think everything good comes to an end and we will have to end this session and the meeting but, of course, we will be able to talk freely the rest of the day. Thank you very much Jerry.

Index